RADIO—Robots in Assisted Living

Vangelis Karkaletsis · Stasinos Konstantopoulos
Nikolaos S. Voros · Roberta Annicchiarico
Maria Dagioglou · Christos P. Antonopoulos
Editors

RADIO—Robots in Assisted Living

Unobtrusive, Efficient, Reliable and Modular Solutions for Independent Ageing

Springer

Editors
Vangelis Karkaletsis
Institute of Informatics
and Telecommunications,
NCSR "Demokritos"
Aghia Paraskevi
Greece

Stasinos Konstantopoulos
Institute of Informatics
and Telecommunications,
NCSR "Demokritos"
Aghia Paraskevi
Greece

Nikolaos S. Voros
Embedded System Design and Application
Lab, Department of Computer
and Informatics Engineering
Technological Educational Institute
of Western Greece
Patras
Greece

Roberta Annicchiarico
Clinical and Behavioral Neurology
Laboratory
IRCCS Fondazione Santa Lucia
Rome
Italy

Maria Dagioglou
Institute of Informatics
and Telecommunications,
NCSR "Demokritos"
Aghia Paraskevi
Greece

Christos P. Antonopoulos
Embedded System Design and Application
Lab, Department of Computer
and Informatics Engineering
Technological Educational Institute
of Western Greece
Patras
Greece

ISBN 978-3-030-06408-2 ISBN 978-3-319-92330-7 (eBook)
https://doi.org/10.1007/978-3-319-92330-7

Printed on acid-free paper

This Springer imprint is published by the registered company Springer Nature Switzerland AG
The registered company address is: Gewerbestrasse 11, 6330 Cham, Switzerland

Preface

Recognizing the highly dynamic area of Ambient Assisted Living (AAL) environments and their potentially huge societal and economic impact, the Horizon 2020 programme set a research topic on integrating robotics technologies in AAL environments. The RADIO project approached the topic with an investigation that spanned three technical topics: (a) integrating machine vision and, more generally, robot perception with Smart Home technical capabilities into a health monitoring system; (b) moving machine vision algorithms to hardware-based processing accelerators; and (c) managing and processing the sensitive raw content collected and the health-related information derived from it. But, most importantly, RADIO investigated the interaction between these technical capabilities and the ever-present and ever-pressing need to balance between *what monitoring is medically required*, the *value of health records to medical research* and *what levels of obtrusion these medical requirements justify*.

To elaborate and to avoid the obtrusion of having to use specific devices in order to have data collected, we restricted our sensing equipment to what is useful and desired independently of its monitoring functionality: a robot that helps you find misplaced items and a Smart Home that automates daily chores are nice things to have; if the same hardware can also be used to collect data about the ability to perform activities of daily living, so much the better. Hardware-based processing is a low-power alternative to CPU processing which increases the robot's battery autonomy, but it is also a safeguard for privacy, touching upon questions of ethics, dignity and obtrusiveness: sensitive content is kept safe by immediately processing at the source and directly discarding, without ever storing in any computer. Finally, the distributed management of medical data can offer new opportunities for both medical practice and medical research, without compromising privacy.

We hope that you will enjoy the RADIO book and appreciate the insights it intends to provide in a topic that cuts across the humanities, health, information technology and engineering disciplines.

Aghia Paraskevi, Greece	Vangelis Karkaletsis
Aghia Paraskevi, Greece	Stasinos Konstantopoulos
Patras, Greece	Nikolaos S. Voros
Rome, Italy	Roberta Annicchiarico
Aghia Paraskevi, Greece	Maria Dagioglou
Patras, Greece	Christos P. Antonopoulos

Acknowledgements

The research work that provided the material for this book was carried out during 2015–2018 in the Horizon 2020 RADIO RIA Project (*Robots in assisted living environments:* Unobtrusive, efficient, reliable and modular solutions for independent ageing) funded by the European Commission under the Grant Agreement number 643892.

The guidance and the comments of the Project Officer *Ms. Monika Lanzenberger* and of the external reviewers are highly appreciated.

Contents

About the Editors

Dr. Vangelis Karkaletsis is Research Director and Head of the Software and Knowledge Engineering Lab (SKEL), Institute of Informatics and Telecommunications, NCSR "Demokritos". His research interests are in the areas of big data management, content analysis, natural language interfaces, ontology engineering and personalization. He has organized international summer schools, workshops and conferences. He is currently Director of the MSc program on Data Science, and responsible for the Institute educational activities. He is co-founder of the spin-off company 'i-sieve Technologies' that exploited SKEL research work on online content analysis. He is currently involved in the founding of the new spin-off company NewSum that exploits SKEL technology on multilingual and multi-document summarization. Dr. Karkaletsis coordinated the Radio project.

Dr. Stasinos Konstantopoulos holds an M.Eng. in Computer Engineering (University of Patras, Greece, 1997), an M.Sc. in Artificial Intelligence (Edinburgh University, UK, 1998) and a Ph.D. on machine learning and computational logic (Groningen University, The Netherlands, 2003). He leads *Roboskel*, the robotics activity of the Institute of Informatics and Telecommunications, NCSR "Demokritos". His main research interests are artificial intelligence and computational logic, and their applications to semantic modelling, data management and robot perception. He has published several papers in these fields and is or has been on the program and organizing committees of various international conferences, including chairing the Programme Committee of the 6th Hellenic AI Conference (SETN 2010), Athens, 2010. Dr. Konstantopoulos was the scientific manager of the Radio project.

Dr. Nikolaos S. Voros received his Diploma in Computer and Informatics Engineering, in 1996, and his Ph.D. degree, in 2001, from University of Patras, Greece. His research interests fall in the area of embedded system design, and include specification techniques for complex embedded telecommunication systems, hardware–software co-design, formal refinement techniques and reuse practices. Currently, Dr. Voros is Assistant Professor at Technological Institute of

Western Greece, Department of Computer and Informatics Engineering where he is leading the Embedded Systems Lab. He was the General Chair of the IEEE Computer Society Annual Symposium on VLSI, which took place in Kefalonia, Greece on July 2010, Program Co-chair for 24th International Conference on Field Programmable Logic and Applications (FPL 2014), which will take place at Technical University of Munich on September 2–4, 2014 and General Chair of the 14th International Symposium on Applied Reconfigurable Computing (ARC 2018) held on May 2–4, Santorini, Greece, 2018. He has served as Associate Editor at IEEE Consumer Electronic Magazine, IEEE Transactions on Nanotechnology, ACM Transactions, Transactions on Reconfigurable Technology and Systems.

Dr. Roberta Annicchiarico is a geriatrician. She has a degree in Medicine (1994) and specialization in Geriatrics (1998) at "La Sapienza" University of Rome; Ph.D. in "Neurosciences, Rehabilitation and Behavioural Sciences" (2003) at "La Sapienza" University of Rome. Since 2002, she is Medical Assistant at Fondazione Santa Lucia, Rome. She is contracted professor of Internal Medicine with focus on Geriatrics at the School of Physiotherapy since 2004 and at the School of Nursing since 2005 (University of Tor Vergata, Rome). She is teacher at the postgraduate courses on "Alzheimer's disease and Dementias", held by Fondazione Santa Lucia since 2001, and was teacher at the "European Master Degree in Preventive and Adapted Physical Activity" (2003). She has been involved in several European Projects. Her main research interests are the disability correlates of chronic diseases, and possible clinical applications of new technologies. Dr. Annicchiarico was the clinical manager of the RADIO Project.

Dr. Maria Dagioglou studied Electrical and Computer Engineering (Democritus University of Thrace, Xanthi, Greece, 2007). She also holds an M.Sc. in Biomedical Engineering (TU Delft, The Netherlands, 2010). During her M.Sc. thesis, she collaborated with the Department of Neuroscience of Erasmus Medical Centre. She was then employed as a Marie Curie Fellow (2010–2013, ITN "C7: Cerebellar-Cortical Control: Cells, Circuits, Computation, and Clinic"), in the Predictive Sensory Motor (PRISM) Lab of the School of Psychology in the University of Birmingham, UK, where she studied on human motor control and learning. She received her Ph.D. in Psychology in July 2014. Since April 2014, she is a research associate at NCSR-D working on autonomous robotic navigation and human–robot interaction. Dr. Dagioglou was the biomedical engineer of the Radio project, coordinating work between the clinical partners and the technical partners.

Dr. Christos P. Antonopoulos received his Diploma and Ph.D. at Electrical Engineering and Computer Technology from the Department of Electrical Engineering and Computer Technology, University of Patras Greece in 2002 and 2008 respectively. From 2002, he has been involved in more than 10 European projects (FP5,6,7 and Horizon 2020) and more than 5 Greek National research projects holding key positions both technical as well as managerial. He has published high number (>65) of research papers and 13 book chapters in international journals and conferences which have received over 450 citations while he has served as editor to two Springer books. From 2002, he has worked as adjunct assistant professor at the Technological Institute of Patras, while from 2010, he is working as adjunct assistant professor at the Computer and Informatics Engineering Department, Technological Educational Institute of Western Greece (Antirio). His main research interests lay in the areas of CyberPhysical Systems, Internet of Things and Ambient Assisted Living Platforms. More specifically, his technical expertise lay in the fields of Wireless Networks, Network Communication Protocols, Network Simulation, Performance Evaluation, Embedded Software, Sensor Networks, Wireless Broadband Access Networks, Embedded System Architecture and Programming. In Radio, Dr. Antonopoulos led the work package that developed the ADL recognition methods.

Chapter 1
Introduction to the RADIO Project

Vangelis Karkaletsis, Stasinos Konstantopoulos and Nikolaos S. Voros

1.1 Introduction

Demographic and epidemiologic transitions have brought a new health care paradigm with the presence of both growing elderly population and chronic diseases [1]. Life expectancy is increasing as well as the need for long-term care. Institutional care for the aged population faces economical struggles with low staffing ratios and consequent quality problems [2, 3].

Although the aforementioned implications of ageing impose societal challenges, at the same time technical advancements in ICT, including robotics, bring new opportunities for the ageing population of Europe, the healthcare systems, as well as the European companies providing relevant technology and services at the global scale. The full realization of this technological potential depends on:

- Concrete evidence for the *benefits for all stakeholders*, including the elderly primary end-users and their formal and informal caregivers (secondary end-users), as well as the healthcare system.
- *Safety of and acceptability by* the end-users.
- *Cost-effectiveness* in acquisition and maintenance, *reliability*, and *flexibility* in being able to meet a range of needs and societal expectations.
- The provision of functionalities that can *reduce admissions and days spent in care institutions*, and prolong the *time spent living in own home.*

V. Karkaletsis (✉) · S. Konstantopoulos
Institute of Informatics and Telecommunications, NCSR “Demokritos”,
Aghia Paraskevi, Greece
e-mail: vangelis@iit.demokritos.gr

N. S. Voros
Embedded System Design and Application Lab,
Computer and Informatics Engineering Department,
Technological Educational Institution of Western Greece, Patras, Greece

V. Karkaletsis et al. (eds.), *RADIO–Robots in Assisted Living*,
https://doi.org/10.1007/978-3-319-92330-7_1

In RADIO, we developed an ***integrated smart home/assistant robot system***, pursuing ***a novel approach to acceptance and unobtrusiveness***: a system where sensing equipment is not discrete but an ***obvious and accepted part of the user's daily life***. By using the integrated smart home/assistant robot system as the sensing equipment for health monitoring, we mask the *functionality* of the sensors rather than the sensors themselves. In this manner, sensors do not need to be discrete and distant or masked and cumbersome to instal; they do however need to be perceived as a natural component of the smart home/assistant robot functionalities.

1.2 Project Objectives

RADIO pursued a novel approach to user acceptance and unobtrusiveness, developing and integrating robotics and home automation technologies that accommodate users' daily living needs, while assuming interaction with the users as an opportunity for clinical monitoring. In this manner, clinical monitoring sensors do not need to be hidden but become an obvious, yet discrete and accepted, part of the user's daily life.

In pursuing this, the project's initial technical objective was to develop methods for recognizing Activities of Daily Living (ADL) and mood which indicate early symptoms of cognitive impairment, frailty, and social exclusion. A further objective was to integrate these methods into the RADIO Home, a system based on existing reliable, safe and low-cost robotics and home automation solutions. Finally, the hardware sensing and processing components of the RADIO Home form a modular system that can be deployed in different configurations and mixes of components without requiring extensive effort or specialized knowledge for reconfiguration. RADIO also envisages to integrate multiple RADIO Home deployments, medical institutions and informal caregivers into an information management and sharing ecosystem that is by design scalable, secure and privacy-preserving.

In developing and evaluating these technologies, RADIO emphasizes how well the RADIO-provided information can serve its clinical monitoring purpose, how it can be easily reconfigured for different environments and end-users satisfying their individual medical needs and sense of privacy and obtrusiveness, and, finally how usable it is and especially by elderly people.

1.3 Overview of RADIO Outcomes

The clinical requirements of the system were defined based on the interRAI assessment system, a set of comprehensive and standardized geriatric assessment tools for institutional and home settings. RADIO analysed the machine perception state of the art in order to establish which interRAI items can be automatically recognized reliably enough to be useful and what sensor data is needed for these perception technologies. Besides technical feasibility and privacy concerns with respect to the sensor data needed, RADIO carried out a more general discussion on obtrusiveness and how it balances with clinical monitoring requirements.

Clinical and unobtrusiveness requirements guided the design of the RADIO architecture, including the inventory of sensors and perception technologies that RADIO develops and integrates as well as the configurability and modularity of the design. What is stressed in the architecture is the modularity of the design, so that the system can adapt to different environments and to different individual clinical needs and perception of obtrusiveness.

Based on this architectural design, RADIO developed ADL and mood recognition methods that analyse a variety of raw data including audiovisual data, range scans and text from social media interactions. RADIO also developed and integrated methods for localizing people and objects in the environment based on Bluetooth Low Energy (BLE) beacons, people identification and home automation device usage. This inventory of elementary methods will be fused into high-level recognition systems. The methods are physically instantiated on the robot's on-board computer, on FPGA implementations or on off-board Raspberry Pi devices. Together with the home automation sensors, this system of processing units creates a heterogeneous wireless networking environment including ZWave and BLE sensors and WiFi sensors and processors. RADIO investigated both the bridging and the communication robustness of this heterogeneous wireless network.

The RADIO Robot prototype and the integrated RADIO Home prototype were finalized and underwent extensive piloting at Asil Hospital, Granollers, Spain and at multiple private homes in Patras, Greece, serviced by Frontida Zois. Regarding usability, both the primary users and caregivers showed a positive attitude towards the RADIO system. Regarding the medical efficacy of the system and the reliability of the measurements, the results were also very positive, especially at the more structured and meticulously prepared piloting room at Granollers. At the Patras trials, the actual deployment and configuration procedure were also part of the testing, aiming to also measure usability from the perspective of the installation and maintenance technician. The system was proven to be possible to instal within one working day in most cases, with few extremely adversarial environments and hardware or network failures hampering installation and operation.

Finally, RADIO proved the concept of connecting RADIO Homes and medical institutions into the RADIO Ecosystem, adding value to the health data collected by RADIO Homes by making it available not only for medical monitoring but also for medical research. Specifically, RADIO developed network security and access control guidelines for direct access to health data by the competent medical personnel, as well as the RASSP protocol for the privacy-preserving mining of the data collected in each Home's database. These expose appropriate programmatic interfaces, so that, and depending on one's access and use case, individual data and time series can be visualized to monitor particular end-users and statistical data aggregations can be visualized or used by R programs to carry out medical research.

1.4 Conclusion

In the previous sections, we presented a brief overview of RADIO project, where its main challenges and perspectives have been analysed. Although the major contributions of RADIO have been described, we have intentionally avoided providing too many technical details. The rationale is that the specific book chapter intends to introduce the main concepts behind RADIO project and not presenting them in detail.

For the latter, the subsequent book chapters provide all the necessary information both for medical and ICT experts. For that purpose, the rest of the book is divided in three main parts. **Part I**: *Early Detection of Emerging Functional Impairments* where the medical experts of RADIO provide insight to functional impairments, **Part II**: *The RADIO System*, where the RADIO technology is presented in detail and **Part III**: *The Road to Commercialization* where the commercialization perspectives of RADIO technology are presented.

References

1. Busso, C., Deng, Z., Yildirim, S., Bulut, M., Lee, C. M., Kazemzadeh, A., et al. (2004). Analysis of emotion recognition using facial expressions, speech and multimodal information. In *Proceedings of the 6th international Conference on Multimodal Interfaces* (pp. 205–211). ACM.
2. Kash, B. A., Hawes, C., & Phillips, C. D. (2007). Comparing staffing levels in the online survey certification and reporting (OSCAR) system with the medicaid cost report data: are differences systematic? *Gerontologist, 47*(4), 480–489.
3. Weech-Maldonado, R., Meret-Hanke, L., Neff, M. C., & Mor, V. (2004). Nurse staffing patterns and quality of care in nursing homes. *Health Care Management Review, 29*(2), 107–116.

Part I
Early Detection of Emerging Functional Impairments

Chapter 2
A System of Recognition Services for Clinical Assessment

Theodoros Giannakopoulos, Stasinos Konstantopoulos, Georgios Siantikos and Vangelis Karkaletsis

2.1 Introduction

As smart, interconnected sensing devices are becoming ubiquitous, more applications are becoming possible by re-arranging and re-connecting sensing and sensor signal analysis in different pipelines. This appears to imply that the finer the grain of the distinct and referenceable services the better, since finer grain allows maximal flexibility; in reality however, there are composite services that make more sense than their components as the finest grain that is exposed. The reasons vary ranging from technical to privacy, to business considerations, but the effect is that systems of services need to be properly designed to assume a satisfactory position between being too fine and too coarsely grained. We shall focus hereon detecting *Activities of Daily Life (ADL)* in a smart home setting. Such a setting offers itself naturally to medical applications and especially independent living applications, where ADL log scan establishes patterns and identifies deviations. These can range from the time spent out of the house or carrying out a given activity, to sleeping patterns, to recognizing whether the user has changed clothes, washed, or other crucial indications required by the medical condition that necessitates monitoring.

To motivate our work, let us assume as an example a general-purpose acoustic feature extraction component that can provide input for different classification engines and models. For our application, we have established that we will detect acoustic events using an SVN engine and that there is no further component that

This chapter is a reprint of 'Design for a System of Multimodal Interconnected ADL Recognition Services' in *Components and services for IoT platforms: Paving the way for IoT standards*, Springer, September 2016.

T. Giannakopoulos · S. Konstantopoulos · G. Siantikos · V. Karkaletsis (✉)
Institute of Informatics and Telecommunications, NCSR "Demokritos",
Aghia Paraskevi, Greece
e-mail: vangelis@iit.demokritos.gr

V. Karkaletsis et al. (eds.), *RADIO–Robots in Assisted Living*,
https://doi.org/10.1007/978-3-319-92330-7_2

needs these features. In this situation, it makes sense to encapsulate the audio acquisition component, the feature extraction component, and the SVN engine under a single acoustic event detection service and not provide an interface for the acoustic features or, even more so, for the audio signal. We have based our decision on the observation that we re-analyse the lower level feature extraction output into a higher level acoustic event output that is more informative and more straightforward to be consumed by other services. Let us now assume that we later decide to apply a fusion algorithm that combines audio and vision. The extracted audiovisual events represent the same real-world events as the acoustic and visual events that they fuse, except that they are associated with a higher confidence and/or carry more attributes than either. In such a situation, our previous decision to bundle acoustic event extraction as a single service and not as an extraction–classification pipeline restricts us to event-level fusion and makes it impossible to apply feature-level fusion algorithms. On the other hand, if we were to use event-level fusion anyway, the finer grained feature-level services would be unnecessary overheads.

Naturally, real-world scenarios are bound to be even more complex. To give another example, consider a system for our ADL monitoring application that comprises the following components:

- Waking up and getting out of bed is recognized in the depth modality
- Moving around the house is tracked in the depth modality
- Moving around the house is tracked and the person moving is identified in the image modality.

In this scenario, subsequent fused image/depth analysis both confirms and adds attributes (the identity of the person) to the original getting-out-of-bed event. A system that measures the time it takes to transfer out of bed will need both the onset of the first event and the subsequent supporting information. However, this system of analysis components cannot be tried under a single service that log the bed *transfer* ADL, since movement tracking will also be useful for logging numerous other activities.

Further applications can also be envisaged, such as proactively offering automations that are relevant to the current ADL context. The design of this application as an extension of a medical monitoring application is straightforward, since it is based on analysing high-level ADL logs. Other applications, however, might require more concrete data and, thus, more flexibility regarding the components of the architecture that they will need to access. In general, the choice of how to best wrap the analysis components and pipelines of such components balances between micro-services that expose thin slices of functionality and heavier services that wrap larger subsystems. Naturally, there can be no ideal solution and each application must use its own requirements to explore the design space. ADL recognition is based on the recognition of events in (possibly multiple) audiovisual signals and on heuristics that characterize sequences or other compositions of events as more abstract ADL events.

In this chapter, we first present the audiovisual sensors and corresponding recognition methods that are typically used in our application domain. By studying the components that make up these methods and the kinds of information exchanges between them, we propose a conceptual architecture. The purpose of our architecture is to integrate existing components developed in different contexts (robotics and the Internet of things) and to make efficient use of processing and transmission resources. To achieve this, we establish articulation points and specify the kind of information that is exchanged at these points. The key design aim is that the architecture applies to the pipelines commonly proposed in the multimodal processing literature and that it clarifies the content and information requirements of the components of these pipelines.

2.2 Audio-Based Event Recognition

Acoustic analysis pipelines include signal acquisition, acoustic feature extraction, and classification of the features into acoustic events. In particular, the following components are typically included in acoustic analysis pipelines:

1. audio acquisition: uses the audio signal to produce a stream of short-term audio frames
2. short-term feature extraction: uses an audio frame to produce a frame feature vector
3. midterm feature extraction: aggregates multiple frame feature vectors into a midterm segment feature vector
4. audio pattern analysis: uses frame and segment feature vectors to produce an event recognition.

In this section, we will present these components and related design choices based on our ADL recognition application.

2.2.1 Feature Extraction

Audio acquisition is based on the cross-platform, open-source PortAudio library [1]. Audio acquisition divides the audio signal into a stream of short-term windows (frames), and short-term features are extracted in an online mode from each frame

Index	Name	Description
1	Zero crossing rate	The rate of sign changes of the signal during the duration of a particular frame
2	Energy	The sum of squares of the signal values, normalized by the respective frame length

(continued)

(continued)

Index	Name	Description
3	Entropy of energy	The entropy of subframes' normalized energies. It can be interpreted as a measure of abrupt changes
4	Spectral centroid	The centre of gravity of the spectrum
5	Spectral spread	The second central moment of the spectrum
6	Spectral entropy	Entropy of the normalized spectral energies for a set of subframe
7	Spectral flux	The squared difference between the normalized magnitudes of the spectra of the two successive frames
8	Spectral rolloff	The frequency below which 90% of the magnitude distribution of the spectrum is concentrated
9–21	MFCCs	Mel Frequency Cepstral Coefficients form a cepstral representation where the frequency bands are not linear but distributed according to the mel scale
22–33	Chroma vector	A 12-element representation of the spectral energy where the bins represent the 12 equal-tempered pitch classes of western-type music (semitone spacing)
34	Chroma deviation	The standard deviation of the 12 chroma coefficients

Short-term feature extraction produces a stream of feature vectors of 34 elements (see Table above) where each vector is calculated from one frame. The time-domain features (features 1–3) are directly extracted from the raw signal samples. The frequency-domain features (features 4–34, apart from the MFCCs) are based on the magnitude of the Discrete Fourier Transform (DFT). Finally, the cepstral domain (e.g. used by the MFCCs) results after applying the Inverse DFT on the logarithmic spectrum. These features and the effect of short-term windowing in audio classification have been discussed in more detail by Kim et al. [2] and Giannakopoulos et al. [3, 4]. What is important to note is that the frame size and the selected features depend on each other, so that a different frame stream, using different frame size, would need to be produced for a different short-term feature extraction component. This observation suggests a very strong coupling between audio acquisition and short-term feature extraction. Furthermore, short-term feature extraction results in a drastically smaller stream than the original audio signal, so that there is also a communications overhead advantage in only providing the short-term feature stream as a service without exposing the audio signal.

2.2.2 *Audio Feature Aggregation*

Another common technique in audio analysis is the processing of the feature sequence on a midterm basis, according to which the audio signal is first divided into midterm windows (segments). For each segment, *midterm feature extraction* uses the short-term feature vector stream to produce a stream of feature statistics, such as the average value of the ZCR (Feature 1). Therefore, each midterm segment is represented by a set of statistics.

2.2.3 Audio Recognition

The final stage is the analysis of patterns in the short and midterm features to infer event annotations. Two types of *audio pattern analysis* are performed:

- *Supervised* A set of predefined classifiers is trained and used to extract respective labels regarding events [3, 5]. Apart from general audio events regarding activities (ADLs), mood extraction is achieved by applying regression and classification methods trained on speech-based emotion recognition data.
- *Unsupervised* Apart from predefined taxonomies of audio events and activities, audio features are used in the context of a clustering procedure, according to which the extracted labels are not known a priori. A typical example is *speaker diarization* or *speaker clustering*, the task of determining who spoke when [6].

For both types for audio pattern analysis, a decision is made for each short-term feature vector taking into account a combined short-term and midterm feature vector. In a sense, the midterm features provide a context within with the short-term features are interpreted. The signal energy, for example, is more informative when combined with the average energy in order to detect clangs and bangs even in overall noisy environments as sudden spikes above the average. Typical values of the midterm segment size can be from 200 ms to several seconds depending on the events that are being recognized. Segments can be overlapping, using a different sliding midterm feature vector with each short-text feature vector, or non-overlapping, using the same midterm feature vector throughout the duration of the segment.

Depending on the technical characteristics of the middleware used, some communication overheads can be reduced by keeping the same midterm feature vector latched to the bus so that it can be read multiple times by the audio pattern analysis component. This potential gain is, however, relatively small as the information to be communicated has been reduced to 34 floating-point features, i.e. 136 bytes. Furthermore, different event recognizers often work better with different segment sizes, so that multiple (typically two or three) midterm feature vectors need to be made available to audio pattern analysis. These observations suggest that there is little optimization value in non-overlapping segments, and that the (more accurate) rolling segments should be preferred. This still leaves open the question of whether midterm feature vectors should be bundled together with the acquisition/short-term feature extraction components as a complete audio feature extraction service, bundled together with the audio pattern analysis components, or provided as an independent service or services (for different segment sizes).

2.3 Recognizing Events in Visual Content

Visual information is recorded through a depth camera, therefore two types of information are adopted in this context: colour video and depth video. Both types of visual information are fed as input to a workflow of visual analytics whose purpose is to extract:

1. activities of daily living (ADLs): a predefined set of events related to ADLs
2. measures related to the user's ability to perform these ADLs (Fig. 2.1).

2.3.1 *Preprocessing*

In our application area, stereoscopic or structured light visual sensors are used to provide both colour and 3D depth information channels. Both channels are

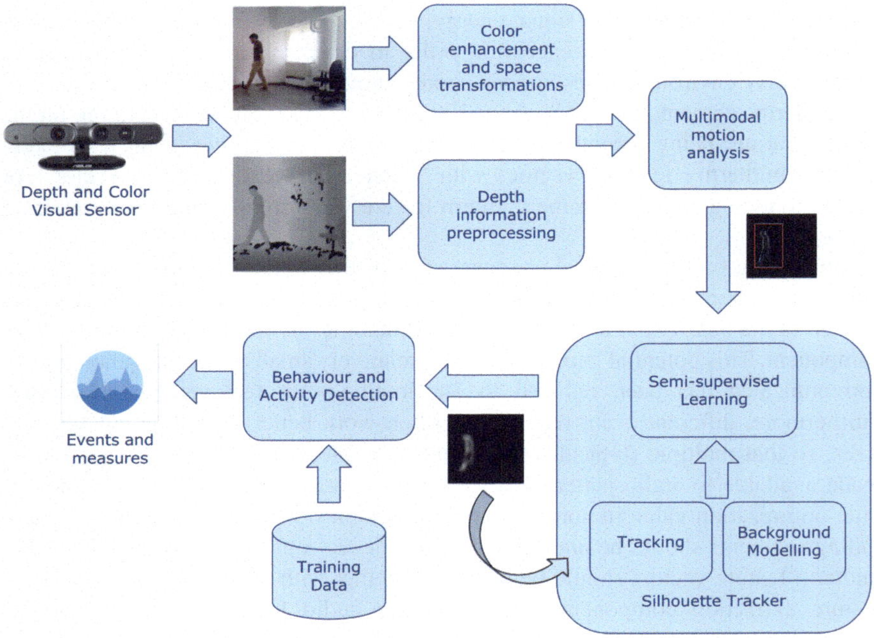

Fig. 2.1 Depth and colour visual analytics workflow

preprocessed in order to provide better representations of the scene. Colour is transformed and normalized in order to achieve colour consistency and lighting conditions independence. In addition, de-noising and hole removal are applied on each depth frame in order to provide the next steps with smoother depth representations.

2.3.2 *Motion Detection*

This submodule aims to function as a triggering functionality for initializing the visual analytics workflow but also as a baseline estimator of the user's spatial information. The adoption of motion detection as a separate submodule is twofold: (a) to enhance the performance of the next visual analytics steps (e.g. make the background estimation more robust) and (b) to minimize the computational complexity of the whole visual workflow by triggering the respective submodules only when necessary.

Motion detection is capable of checking the existence of motion within the visual information. For each processing time unit (i.e. video frame), a single thresholding rule is adopted for extra low computational complexity, in order to infer the existence of motion. If no motion is detected, then the background model is updated as described in the next paragraph. For better performance, separate channels are used in order to estimate the motion of each frame: depth-based distance metrics along with three different colour space distance metrics. A simple weighted average fusion approach is used to generate the final two-dimensional distance metric that is used in the thresholding criterion that detects the motion area. The result of this procedure is a bounding box of the motion area.

Before combining the different modalities, it is important to note that visual *registration* is applied, in order to align the different representations of the same scene into one common spatial representation. Especially between the depth and colour channels, it is very important to apply such geometric transformations, since the two channels are heavily misaligned on most sensors.

2.3.3 *Silhouette Tracking*

The goal of this submodule is to detect and track the exact positions of the pixels associated to the person's silhouette. Towards this end, the following algorithmic stages are adopted:

- Background modelling: The goal here is to estimate a statistical model that describes the background of the visual information, so that it is subtracted in the main visual analysis steps. The background subtraction submodule is triggered from the motion detection service as described in the previous paragraph. As soon as the module is triggered, the following steps are executed:

  - the detected as 'motion' frames are captured to memory
  - contrast and light normalization is applied to remove unwanted dependencies
  - gamma correction is applied
  - the background model is extracted using the MOG operator [7]
  - the outline of foreground objects is finally estimated using a set of morphological operations [8].

- Tracking: The goal of this step is to model the moving object's dynamics in order to track the exact position of the user.
- Semisupervised Learning: At each stage, a clustering algorithm is applied based on the current estimated background, the feedback from the tracking algorithm as well as the raw depth info of the current frame, in order to decide on the final silhouette estimate.

2.3.4 *Behaviour and Activity Detection*

Given the position and exact shape of the user's silhouette, a series of supervised and unsupervised machine learning approaches is applied in order to:

- extract a set of predefined activities (stand up, sitting, lying in bed, walking, running, eating, etc.). Towards this end, annotated data are used to train the respective classifiers.
- extract body key points using supervised models.
- detect faces and extract facial features. Also, if provided, the supervised database stores facial features of known users and the respective module also extract user ID (identification).
- extract clothing-related information (i.e. if the user has changed clothes since her last appearance on the sensor) [9].
- estimate metrics related to the user's ability to walk. Towards this end, unsupervised temporal modelling is adopted as the means to extract measures that quantify the gait: average speed, time required to walk four metres, etc.

2.3.5 *Fused Audiovisual Analysis*

Apart from the audio and visual workflows that extract respective high-level information and metadata regarding activities and measures, the early and late fusion approaches are used to extract information from the combined audio and visual modalities. One example is combining facial features with acoustic features in the context of a speaker diarization method that extracts user labels based on speech and facial cues [10]. In this *early fusion* example, the acoustic and visual feature vectors are fused. By contrast, late fusion approaches are used for behaviour recognition. In particular, multimodal events can be recognized by combining events in each modality that represent the same physical event.

2.4 ADL Recognition Architecture

Based on our analysis of the ADL recognition methods described, we will now proceed to bundle the relevant components into services and to specify these services' information outputs and requirements. These services will be used as the building blocks of our ADL recognition architecture in this section. Our usage scenario is set in an assisted living environment with static sensors and a mobile robot which acts as a mobile sensing platform. In this setting, the clinical requirement is to monitor activities of daily life in order to report aggregated logs about the occurrence of specific ADLs, signs of physical activity, as well as performance measurements such as time needed to get off the bed or to walk a given distance [11]. In our design, we foresee acoustic sensors that integrate a microphone with Raspberry Pi, the RADIO Robot that integrates microphone, depth and colour camera and on-board computer (Chap. 6), and an off-board computer that acts as the gateway to the home and the orchestrator of the overall monitoring and reporting. This physical infrastructure is used to deploy the sensing services and the ADL recognition services that use them.

There is a single acoustic features interface which publishes a stream of triplets of feature vectors. Each message in the stream contains the current short-term frame feature vector and two midterm rolling averages of different numbers of frames to accommodate analyses that require deeper or more shallow acoustic contexts. This interface was chosen because at our 50 Hz frame rate volume of traffic generated by three floating-point feature vectors is insignificant and this interface lifts the requirement to have a middleware that can latch midterm feature vectors or synchronize midterm and short-term feature vectors. Exposing the complete acquisition feature extraction pipeline as a single service also allows us to provide a unified acoustic feature service over two heterogeneous implementations [12]:

- The TurtleBot2 implementation comprises a microphone device driver and a feature extraction component that communicate using the ROS middleware. The Robot Operating System (ROS) is a set of software libraries and tools for developing distributed applications in robotics; please cf. http://www.ros.org for more details. The service end point is a bridge that simultaneously connects to the robot-internal ROS middleware and to the home WiFi to access robot-external services.
- The Raspberry implementation comprises a microphone device driver and a feature extraction component that communicate using MQTT, which is an

extremely lightweight publish—subscribe messaging middleware for the Internet of Things; please cf. http://mqtt.org for more details. The service end point is a bridge that simultaneously connects to MQTT and to the home WiFi to access external services.

All instances of the acoustic features service push their vector streams to the audio pattern analysis service. This service implements unsupervised and (previously trained) supervised machine learning methods that recognize ADL events from acoustic feature vectors. The audio pattern analysis service is also distributed, with instances executing at the Raspberry and the robot's computer. The vision sensing components are analogously implemented as image acquisition, feature extraction, and pattern recognition services. One divergence from the acoustic analysis case is that the graph of dependencies between vision services is not a linear progression from the content to more abstract features and events: motion detection is the only service that constantly consumes features and it triggers more complex analyses as soon as motion is detected. Furthermore, there is no single feature set that is used by all visual analyses and analyses are occasionally stacked more deeply that the features/events/ADLs layers of acoustic ADL detection. The services and interfaces design described here is also depicted in Fig. 2.2.

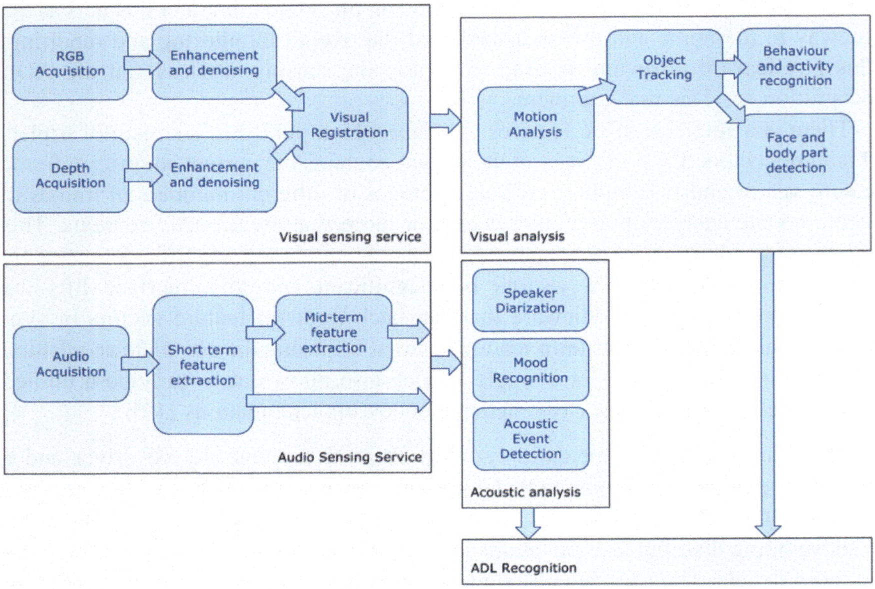

Fig. 2.2 Conceptual architecture of audiovisual analysis

2.5 Conclusion

We presented a system of services that interact to recognize ADLs from audiovisual sensors. Our design integrates subsystems which were originally integrated using heterogeneous middleware infrastructures. We have proposed articulation points for re-structuring these existing pipelines into a new set of services. In order to establish the right level of granularity for the functionality bundled under a single service, we used common patterns in the audiovisual analysis literature to identify services that would practically never need to be broken down into finer services.

The most prominent future research direction is the dynamic handling of early fusion methods. For such methods, the recognition component must have access to both the acoustic and the visual features. In our current design, this is not as issue as in the only situation where this is necessary (scenes captures by the robot) both sensors happen to be on the same ROS middleware and the audiovisual features can be easily consumed by the same component. As this will not be the case in general, our plan is to transfer concepts and technologies from the distributed processing literature. Although developed to address different problems (namely, processing large scale data), transferring such technologies to our application will allow us to develop distributed fusion components. In this manner, an early fusion component can perform calculations over distributed feature vectors without requiring that they are collected at a single computation node, applying the communication overhead optimizations developed by the distributed computation community to minimize the communication of intermediate results.

Another future research direction pertains to incorporating speech recognition in the system. Speech recognition uses radically different features than those computed for acoustic processing. Naturally, one can always concatenate or interleave the feature vectors produced for acoustic and speech processors in order to accommodate both. It is, however, worth investigating whether a study of the feature extraction methods proposed in the speech recognition literature can reveal opportunities for a more efficient integration of the acoustic and speech feature extraction components.

References

1. Bencina, R., & Burk, P. (2001). PortAudio—an open source cross platform audio API. In *Proceedings of the International Computer Music Conference*, Havana (pp. 263–266).
2. Kim, H. G., Moreau, N., & Sikora, T. (2006). *MPEG-7 audio and beyond: Audio content indexing and retrieval*. Hoboken, NJ: Wiley.
3. Giannakopoulos, T (2015). pyAudioAnalysis: An open-source Python library for audio signal analysis. *PloS One, 10*(12).
4. Giannakopoulos, T., & Pikrakis, A. (2014). *Introduction to audio analysis: A MATLAB approach*. Academic Press.

5. Siantikos, G., Sgouropoulos, D., Giannakopoulos, T., & Spyrou, E. (2015). Fusing multiple audio sensors for acoustic event detection. In *Proceedings of the 9th International Symposium on Image and Signal Processing and Analysis (ISPA 2015)* (pp. 265–269). IEEE.
6. Giannakopoulos, T., & Petridis, S. (2015). Fisher linear semi-discriminant analysis for speaker diarization. *IEEE Transactions on Audio, Speech, and Language Processing, 20*(7).
7. KaewTraKulPong, P., & Bowden, R. (2002). An improved adaptive background mixture model for real-time tracking with shadow detection. In *Video-based surveillance systems* (pp. 135–144). Berlin: Springer.
8. Sgouropoulos, D., Spyrou, E., Siantikos, G., & Giannakopoulos, T. (2015). Counting and tracking people in a smart room: An IoT approach. In *Proceedings of the 10th International Workshop on Semantic and Social Media Adaptation and Personalization (SMAP 2015)*. IEEE.
9. Sgouropoulos, D., Giannakopoulos, T., Siantikos, G., Spyrou, E., & Perantonis, S. (2014). Detection of clothes change fusing color, texture, edge and depth information. In *E-Business and Telecommunications* (pp. 383–392). Berlin: Springer.
10. Sarafianos, N., Giannakopoulos, T., & Petridis, S. (2014). Audio-visual speaker diarization using Fisher linear semi-discriminant analysis. *Multimedia Tools and Applications*, 1–16.
11. *RADIO project: Deliverable 2.2: Early detection methods and relevant system requirements*. Tech. Rep. (2015). http://radio-project.eu/deliverables.
12. Siantikos, G., Giannakopoulos, T., & Konstantopoulos, S. (2016). A low-cost approach for detecting activities of daily living using audio information: A use case on bathroom activity monitoring. In *Proceedings of the 2nd International Conference on Information and Communication Technologies for Ageing Well and e-Health (ICT4AWE 2016)*, Rome, Italy.

Chapter 3
Obtrusiveness Considerations of AAL Environments

S. Ariño Blasco, D. Navarro Llobet and G. Koumanakos

3.1 Introduction

The word *obtrusive* is being used increasingly to describe new technologies, including information technology, automation and robotics. Despite the importance of the attributes of the term obtrusive in these technological fields, there is still no clear definition. The term becomes even more confusing when there are no equivalent terms in other languages and should be introduced as an Anglicism. This term is used as an adjective for something too 'apparent/prominent' with a 'striking' or 'conspicuous' no way acceptable or obstructive manner. It means something undesirably prominent, undesirably bulky. The term can refer to something undesirably prominent physically, psychologically or both.

In relation to the field of ambient assistive living (AAL) environments, obtrusiveness can be related to either hardware or software aspects of the system. In case of a robot or another assistive device, obtrusiveness can be used to describe the occupation of the discreet space of the users, either in physical, mental or psychological form. In other instances, unobtrusiveness is used as a synonym to ease of use, user-friendliness, etc. As pointed out by Hensel [1], obtrusiveness follows four rules: (1) it is the result of an addition of features (multicomponent), (2) it depends where the technology applies, (3) the user will not be the only subject that could be affected but also others living around and (4) it is subjective.

Obtrusiveness depends heavily on the subjective perceptions and the prioritization of needs of each user [2]. Older adults will not adopt a health-related technology if it does not fulfil their current levels of need, such as security and

S. Ariño Blasco · D. Navarro Llobet (✉)
Fundació Privada Hospital Asil de Granollers, Granollers, Spain
e-mail: diananavarro@fhag.es

G. Koumanakos
Frontida Zois, Patras, Greece

V. Karkaletsis et al. (eds.), *RADIO–Robots in Assisted Living*,
https://doi.org/10.1007/978-3-319-92330-7_3

safety, no matter how unobtrusive, smart, affordable or powerful the technology is [3, 4]. Demiris and colleagues conducted a series of focus groups to assess older adults' perceptions and expectations of specific smart home technologies. The results showed that most participants acknowledged the need for a balance between the benefits of monitoring, determined by level of need, and the perceived intrusion into their privacy [5]. Home robots, alone or in combination with a limited set of sensors embedded in the home environment, have the potential to achieve effective monitoring of individuals in a rather unobtrusive way and with very limited likelihood of generating privacy concerns [6].

In order to approach obtrusiveness aspects in a global way, in RADIO we adopted Hensel and colleagues' conceptual framework [1] for the definition of 'obtrusiveness', which is, to our knowledge, the most complete framework so far in this field. In this framework, obtrusiveness is described by eight subcategories. In the following sections of this chapter, we present literature related to each dimension and describe what aspects of the RADIO system are pertinent to each dimension.

3.2 Physical Dimension

The physical dimension of obtrusiveness is related to functional dependence, discomfort or strain, excessive noise, obstruction or impediment in space, aesthetic incongruence [1]. The physical dimension is affected significantly by the morphology of the particular setting where the elderly person lives, and of course by the presence of the equipment as functioning part of this setting. Moreover, in terms of the robot use, excessive noise and proximity to the user during operation must be considered. The issues in RADIO system related to the physical dimension of obtrusiveness concern: the use of environmental (smart home) sensors versus wearable sensors, the existence of a robot and the environment itself (institutional vs. private).

A striking example of physical dimension obtrusiveness is wearable sensors, which can result in discomfort and inconvenience for the users [7]. The form and aesthetics of the device should not affect normal daily behaviour [4]. If not carefully designed, wearable sensors can take a central role in the user's attention and concerns, jeopardizing accuracy and consistency in the measurements [8]. For these reasons, sensors installed in the environment (smart houses), provided that they do not impact on the user's privacy, are an acceptable solution that assumes no extra burden for wearing and maintaining the sensors.

However, elderly people express concerns about the appearance of technology (for the prominence or interference) when they find it in their homes [9]. This highlights the importance of the environmental dimension (home vs. institution) regarding obtrusiveness [1]. Some technologies could be implemented in an institutional scenario because the space in the nursing home is greater than in a private home. Moreover, this is also related to the concept of ownership. This can be phrased as follows: 'In my home I would not like to have obtrusive, prominent things around (because of aesthetics and potential damage), however in the Nursing Home I do not care, it is not my territory'.

Elderly people do not seem to consider a domestic robot equipped with sensors as a possible source of intrusion/disturbance in personal life [10]. Moreover, they show more positive reactions and evaluations when having the opportunity to know what a robot can actually do in the domestic environment. However, discomfort or strain could be experienced when interacting with socially intelligent robots. A relevant survey [11] showed that the majority of the subjects disliked the robot moving behind them, blocking their path or moving on collision path towards them. The majority of subjects experienced discomfort when the robot was performing a task within the social zone reserved for human–human face-to-face conversations (closer than 3 m). Proximity between the robot and the user raises substantial questions about safety, and that is why safety and dependability of the physical interaction have to be evaluated considering all the different components of a robot, from mechanisms to actuators, and from sensing to control [12].

3.3 Usability Dimension

The usability dimension of obtrusiveness is related to lack of user-friendliness or accessibility, additional demands on time and effort [1]. ISO 9241[1] guidelines refer to usability as the 'extent to which a product can be used by specified users to achieve specified goals with effectiveness, efficiency and satisfaction in a specified context of use'. In the RADIO environment, the usability of the system (or lack thereof) concerns the interaction between the user and the robot or the smart home via the use of mobile devices (smartphones or tablets). A user-friendly and easy to access graphical user interface (GUI) guarantees uninterrupted interaction with the system and thus sufficient opportunities for monitoring.

The attitude of older people towards technology can be a major constraint regarding the usability of a system. '*Computer anxiety*' can have a significant negative impact on the perceived ease of use and thus on the behaviour and performance of the user [13]. According to Hirsch et al. [14], user perceptions of their own abilities are often out of step with their actual capabilities causing them either to be fearful of attempting relatively safe tasks, or in case of overestimation of their capabilities to undertake risky tasks. On the other hand, Giuliani et al. [15] put under dispute the widespread stereotype that elderly people would be hostile to changes, even more when it comes to the introduction of technological devices. They argue that technological devices clearly go unused only when they appear to be unrealistic or in conflict with the main goal of their action.

[1]ISO 9241 Ergonomics of Human System Interaction, Part 11: Usability: Definitions and concepts

It thus becomes clear that the design of assistive technologies is extremely significant as a factor contributing to disparity between perceived and actual capabilities, promoting easiness of usage. For this reason, it is an absolute priority that the actual needs of stakeholders including end users, caregivers and clinical professionals should be the first to be taken under consideration for the design and implementation of AAL technologies and not the functional capabilities of the technological advancements [16]. Researchers and technology developers are responsible for considering how they will address the needs and limitations of older adults with regard to their interface with technology [17].

Moreover, we also consider in this dimension the notion of utility[2] and usefulness. An important precondition for the elderly to accept the technology is that they are be able to recognize and agree with the benefits it promises to provide [18]. Elderly population demonstrates a priori a less perceived need and limited usefulness of technologies than adult population generally [19]. However, they will adopt a new IT system if they perceive it useful, even if they dislike it. Thus, perceived need and usefulness of the system to maintain independence and prevent being relocated to a more restrictive environment are key to acceptance, and AAL technologies need to be customized to the concerns of the key stakeholders in order to promote adoption and buy-in [20].

Scopeliti et al. [21] found that elderly people in comparison with younger ones are the most fearful at the prospect of having a robot at home, and they try to ward off their anxiety by attributing features to robots like small size, slow motion or feminine voice. They also showed some mistrust towards machines that are likely to be unsafe by preferring to limit the autonomy of the machine, being pre-programmed in a fixed way and not free to move at will inside the house. The same study argues that the mistrust shown by the elderly people is mostly due to an emotional difficulty with technology and absence of stimulation, rather than on a well-founded assessment of how technology can or cannot improve their life.

Appreciating the importance of the usability dimension, RADIO pilot studies explicitly investigated the usability of the RADIO system. More specifically, the formative phase of RADIO pilots tested an existing graphical user interface (GUI) to get feedback on usability requirements for designing RADIO's GUIs. Based on the results, RADIO GUI was designed satisfying several requirements such as larger text fonts, more intense colour contrast and more straightforward navigation though several functions offered. The intermediate and summative phases of RADIO's pilot studies further investigated the usability of the RADIO prototype, regarding aspects of usability of the overall system in two settings (FZ—home environment and FHAG—institutional care) with the engagement of older people from different social and cultural backgrounds.

---

[2] I SO. Ergonomics of human-system interaction. Part 210: Human-centred design for interactive systems. ISO International Standards; 2015; Available from: http://www.iso.org/iso/home/store/catalogue_tc/catalogue_detail.htm?csnumber=52075.

3.4 Privacy Dimension

The privacy dimension concerns not only the invasion of personal information but also the violation of the personal space of home [1]. In RADIO, both of these aspects are relevant and analysed below.

Privacy is considered inherent to the human nature and for this, it has been thoroughly analysed from legal, ethical and philosophical point of view. The first milestone in the legal definition of privacy goes back to 1890 when Warren and Brandeis defined privacy as '*the right to be alone*' that is the right to protect one's private sphere against interferences from others [22]. In 1967, Westin defined privacy as 'the individuals' right to control the circulation of information concerning him or her' [23]. According to Schoeman [24]: '*A person has privacy to the extent that others have limited access to information about him, the intimacies of his life, or his thoughts or his body*'. Rochelandet [25] identified three dimensions of privacy. The first dimension, defined as the secret, is the individual's capacity to control collection and usage of his/her personal data. The second dimension regards the tranquillity or «the right to be left alone» and therefore does concern the accessibility to a person. The third dimension concerns the autonomy, which is the individual capacity to take the decisions for own self.

As technology progresses, the rapidly evolving capacities of AAL systems to monitor, access and store personal data will always be under close and meticulous inspection as to how much they affect the end user's right to privacy. In terms of the research data collection and usage, RADIO strictly complied to the Data Protection Directive (1995/46/EC) and the Privacy and Electronic Communications Directive (2002/58/EC), which were currently addressing data protection, privacy and to a certain extent, security. It should also be noted that the data collection procedure followed during RADIO adhered to strict ethical requirements which suffice to cover the requirement imposed by the new General Data Protection Regulation (GDPR).

In terms of the foreseen management of private data during an eventual production deployment, the RADIO architecture provides two modes of access: aggregated for research purposes and detailed for medical purposes. In aggregated mode, the RADIO system integrates the RASSP Protocol [26] through which statistics that are useful for medical research can be computed over the RADIO users' sensitive data without disclosing individual data points. In the detailed mode, conventional authorization, access control and encrypted transmission protocols are used so that authorized users have access to private data. What should also be stressed is that in either mode of operation, the RADIO system emphasizes that raw audiovisual content is always analysed on-site and immediately discarded, and it is only abstract information that is within the scope of the data management discussed above.

The privacy dimension goes further than the psychological dimension; it points actually to human dignity. This is particularly relevant in the field of measurement techniques throughout external non-wearable sensors because they are undetectable by the subjects. In this regard, we must bring special attention to 'awareness or acceptance of measurement' because without this element of a user's approval, we could violate the privacy or intimacy of the individual. Being 'invisible' does not mean that the subject is not aware that a measurement is being taken.

Regarding the tranquillity and the autonomy, older adults' perceptions of smart home technologies depend on the trade-off between individual preferences and needs. While the continued 24 h/7 days a week monitoring can cause loss of privacy and threaten one's dignity, at the same time, it is as a way to ensure safety and security [27]. This is also extended to the place where monitoring takes place; the most evident example regards monitoring in the bedroom and bathroom, areas where highly private yet risky activities take place [28]. Moreover, the strong aversion to institutionalization and the increased sense of safety and security can result in no concerns related to privacy [4].

The use of assistive robots in the AAL environments also raises issues of privacy, related to both their movement in the private space and their monitoring capabilities (where and what they monitor). However, if the user can control robot's circulation within the living environment, this can safeguard privacy and its use may even be perceived less of a privacy invasion compared to having a caregiver around, especially in potentially embarrassing situations [29]. In case of physically assistive robots, care must also be taken with protocols for touching, something that is a standard part of human caretaker training [30].

3.5 Function Dimension

The function dimension is related to malfunction or suboptimal performance, inaccurate measurement, restriction in distance or time away from home, and perception of lack of usefulness [1]. In the context of RADIO, this dimension is applicable both in the sanity and accuracy of ADL measurements and in the perception of lack of usefulness by its primary and secondary users.

Concerns regarding the usage and functionality of the assisted living devices as well as system reliability are an important issue for all users, and it becomes even more crucial considering the possible frailty and less resilience of an older user [27]. Especially in the home environment, the level of autonomy of the users may threaten—to a lesser or greater extent—their safety.

In a human–robot interaction (HRI) system, suboptimal performance can also come as a failure to complete a task due to the unpredictable nature of the interaction (e.g. unexpected changes of humans' behaviour or preferences). Such failures cannot be ruled out, in principle, but can be managed with suitable policies [12].

3.6 Human Interaction Dimension

This dimension refers to the threat to replace in-person contacts, lack of human response in emergencies and detrimental effects on relationships [1]. In RADIO, this dimension comes relevant because of the presence of the assistive robot.

Human contacts are particularly valued in supporting the ageing process. In general, the need to quickly establish human contact on a daily basis is especially important for elderly people, and caring is an essential factor for enhancing the feeling of security for them [31]. Technology advancements while searching to satisfy the versatile nature of the older people's needs should always leave space for the beneficial contribution of the personal contact either through the physical presence of the caregiver or even through the human–machine interface. In many articles, worries are expressed that the usage of assisted living technology might lead to loss of human contact [28, 32–37]. Thus, the future success of AAL environments will depend in large part on the human–machine interface, where the individual's needs and expectations will be adequately addressed [38]. Technology should be designed with ease of use by older adults, and it should provide opportunities for more social contact. Social contact is a sign of health in older adults, and monitoring systems should be designed with this concern in mind and not as a substitute for skilled caregivers [39].

The loss of human contact and social interaction always comes as a major concern to researchers in HRI. The loss of social interaction can result in increased stress and cognitive decline. It seems that reduced social interaction can have a measurable impact on the health and well-being of the elderly, and reinforces the idea that depriving them of such contact is unethical [40]. Especially in the case of physically assistive robots, where users could be both vulnerable and dependent, the main concerns are as follows: (a) the involvement of robots in particularly intimate activities such as bathing and sanitation, (b) direct physical contact between robots and humans and (c) the high probability of user's forming emotional bonds with robots in environments that otherwise may be lacking in human companionship [30].

Older people have different preferences, between robotics and human assistance, when they have to receive care. In case of personal care tasks and leisure, elder people seem to prefer human caregiving, while they prefer robotics for more basic tasks such as manipulating objects or information management [41, 42]. In various cases, even if people are happy to adopt a new technology and do not feel that it will replace in-person contact, they would still prefer a human response in the case of a crisis [43].

The robot's physical embodiment, form and level of anthropomorphism, and the simplicity or complexity of the design are some of the key research areas needing further attention. Human-like robots might appear 'unnatural' and evoke feelings of repulsion in humans [11]. Cesta et al. [44] reported that elderly people clearly indicated their preference for a faceless robot, hardly resembling a human being, as better integrated into the home setting and more valued as a source of advantages in the management of everyday life. Naturally, robot's image preferences are influenced by the cultural background of the users as well. Nevertheless, the formation of emotional bonds might be inevitable regardless of the morphology of the platform and the direction of the design process towards encouraging or discouraging this [45].

3.7 Self-concept Dimension

This dimension of obtrusiveness is related to symbols of loss of independence, due to embarrassment, or stigma [1]. This construct is closely related to the concept of psychological obtrusiveness. It is interesting that some specific technologies for elderly contain stigmatizing symbols that can backfire at the adoption of these 'gerontotechnologies' [19]. Elderly people feel concern about dependency; their self-esteem is compromised when they reveal assistive aids in public, and they try to avoid the use of those aids in a paradoxical mode. For instance, they are frequent fallers but they are reluctant to use zimmer frames or walking canes. The more prominent the presence of a device is (obtrusiveness), the more negative its symbol is and the greater the impact on self-esteem. Naturally, the RADIO system could trigger feelings of stigmatization as it is a product targeted to elderly.

A significant barrier to technology adoption is the perception elderly people have about themselves and their abilities [21, 27]. The adoption of an assistive or monitoring technology is considered by many an acknowledgement of their frailty, and thus, older adults who might benefit the most from it might be the persons least likely to adopt it [46]. Older adults found it difficult to ask for help and moving from being independent to becoming a service user is considered a life-changing step, strongly associated with the idea of 'giving up' or of admitting defeat [31]. Monitoring devices may cause users to feel ashamed and powerless and pose a stigmatizing aesthetic that leads older people to avoid using them outside their homes or in limited environments because of their embarrassment of being relied on assistive devices [14].

Aesthetic considerations in product design and early adoption of technology can be crucial for the acceptance of assistive systems. The size and form of devices as well as product function and underlying technology are essential components of the assistive technology design. Especially, the minimization of the size and the visibility of a solution are seen as important aspects for reducing stigmatization [35, 36]. Moreover, employing technology before it is actually needed and presenting it as a useful and helpful solution that promotes safety could delay the changes associated with the onset of disability and avoid stigmatizing older persons [39]. This is in line with the fact that the lack of enthusiasm of older people, in contrast to that of their family members, to adopt a monitoring system is presented often as a need for pragmatic justification than as an a priori rejection of the concept [47].

It is true that as elderly people grow old, they constantly assemble and redefine their own attitudes towards ageing. Therefore, the preconceptions of the elderly held by service providers do not correspond to the reality. In reality, fixed conception definitions of the elderly that would embrace all elderly people are impossible [31].

3.8 Routine Dimension

This dimension refers to interference with daily activities and the acquisition of new rituals [1]. Questions relevant to this dimension are whether users have to set up the system (on daily basis) and how this affects their daily life; whether they have to alter their daily schedule (e.g. the waking up time), etc. The RADIO system by design was built to minimize interference with daily routine by excluding from the solution wearable devices, ensuring maximum autonomy of the robot and pursuing monitoring opportunities on the basis of the interaction with the user rather than the on the basis of a predetermined schedule.

Another source of obtrusiveness in terms of interruption of one's routine comes from the automatization of tasks in the context of the smart home, such as the automatic control of lights, temperature, etc. The design and automation of such routine tasks must take into account the level of control retained by the user, which routine tasks can be automated and how user's attention is attracted if necessary for the accomplishment of certain tasks [48].

An alarming issue in the development of smart homes is that of viewing users as dependent patients instead of enhancing their engagement, social inclusion and independence [33]. Again, the design of such environments must be driven primarily by the needs of older adults and not by the features of current technology. Failing to do so can lead to disempowerment of older people and discourage them from staying active, physically and possibly even mentally [49]. The trade-off between assistance and autonomy lies in allowing older people to use their competence. Otherwise, autonomy might negatively impact their self-efficacy, since too much support may lead to a loss of autonomy or even decline of capability [50].

3.9 Sustainability Dimension

The sustainability dimension of obtrusiveness is related to concerns about affordability, future needs and abilities [1]. In other words, it describes the hesitation to make a commitment to a technology that is expensive to acquire and maintain or that might solve only short-term problems but would require a complete replacement to address future needs and abilities. Sustainability dimension is well within the scope of RADIO. Specifically, affordability is one of the core objectives and has influenced several key decisions in system design. Moreover, extensibility for future use cases and needs is also accommodated by establishing software and hardware components that can be reused by other systems to satisfy further clinical requirements pertinent to different medical conditions and user needs.

Monitoring technologies need to be customized to the concerns of the key stakeholders in order to promote adoption and buy-in [20]. There is an obvious shift of the elderly care services from the hospitals to homes, where the provision of the services can be provided more efficiently and tailored to the different needs and particularities of each individual. There is a strong belief that the user-centred, home-based system will become the basis of health care in the future. However, assisted living technological innovations tend to be dominated by suppliers providing a technology push, rather than a demand-pull approach, causing user disappointment resulting from inadequate comprehension of user needs and poor demands for products and services to be used in smart homes [51].

Thus, stakeholder participation is critical to usability and adoption, particularly to accommodate the needs of older adults [52]. Nevertheless, the design method can be a universal design or 'design for all' approach to create barrier-free designs for the widest audience possible while the alternative perspective is that the large degree of variability in the overall health, functional status and cognitive status of older adults precludes such an approach.

Naturally, the cost of any technology is a crucial factor for the adoption of it [13, 18, 27]. Considering the average income of the target population during the design phase and securing financial support from the government or health insurance companies in the uptake phase are both crucial for the diffusion of AAL technologies. Nevertheless, the large-scale implementation of AAL technologies could contribute to cost reduction, allowing them to become available for everyone, and by this annihilating any problems of equity related with the financial capabilities of each user, and the phenomenon of stigmatization [53].

3.10 Obtrusiveness and RADIO Home Visitors

The monitoring of ADLs, especially in a private residence, can be obtrusive not only to the residents but also to their visitors. Interestingly, this highlights the concept of obtrusiveness itself: subjective, multifactorial, environment dependent and multi-target (individual vs. group).

To the best of our knowledge, there is no literature related to this topic. The only relevant information we were able to spot is included in Cortney et al. [43] and actually comments on aesthetic incongruence:

> ...one participant described how distracting she found the assistive technologies in another resident's apartment: '[it] concerned me in M's room when I saw those things [motion sensors]. I thought that would—I would always be looking at them. And they said they could put it up higher on the wall. It's still there. You're still going to look at it'.

From a data privacy perspective, the following directives are related to monitoring by CCTV and phone call recording. Data Protection Directive (95/46/EC) imposes broad obligations on those who collect personal data and confers broad rights on individuals about whom data are collected. Personal data is defined as any information relating to an identified or identifiable natural person [Article 2(a)]. The Directive does not apply to the processing of personal data by a natural person in the course of a purely personal or household activity [Article 3(2)].

3.11 Conclusions

Obtrusiveness is a subjective, multidimensional related to primary users' perceptions, needs and psychology, to functional characteristics of software and hardware components of a system, to clinical requirements as well as sustainability factors. It is obvious from the previous analysis that the different dimensions of obtrusiveness might conflict each other. The magnitude of the obtrusiveness is heavily affected by the self-perception of need of the user, and thus, in each case, it should be examined under the subjective conditions that exist in each user's micro-environment and in accordance to personal perceptions.

As an example, the dimensions of *privacy* and *usability* appear to be weighted by each individual's *self-concept* of need and independence. Elderly might accept a technology with significant privacy implications given its overall value for sustaining a more independent lifestyle [50]. Compromises in privacy are most likely to happen and to be accepted when there is a clear benefit for the users [27]. For instance, the privacy lost from accepting video cameras could only be acceptable if it prevented transfer to a long-term care facility which represents the greatest loss in autonomy [54]. Usability of a given technological infrastructure for elderly people might well be affected by the lack of perceived need as being a reflection of current health status [28]. Moreover, social, emotional and environmental factors can also compromise usability. Elders might reject a device that does not match their environment or makes them feel embarrassed even if it useful for them [14].

For acquiring the best possible result for the users, and for exploiting the full potential of the technology's capacities, it seems very likely that the compromise of some aspects of obtrusiveness for the accomplishment of the best possible safety and monitoring conditions for a user will result in a trade-off between needs and obtrusiveness [40]. It is very important for the assisted living infrastructure to be able to treat obtrusiveness concerns without compromising the quality of the necessary functions and services, and the healthcare principles [55].

References

1. Hensel, B. K., Demiris, G., & Courtney, K. L. (2006). Defining obtrusiveness in home telehealth technologies: A conceptual framework. *Journal of the American Medical Informatics Association, 13*(4), 428–431.
2. McCreadie, C., Tinker, A. (2005). The acceptability of assistive technology to older people. *Ageing & Society, 25*(1), 91–110.
3. Thielke, S., Harniss, M., Thompson, H., Patel, S., Demiris, G., Johnson, K. (2012). Maslow's hierarchy of human needs and the adoption of health-related technologies for older adults. *Ageing International, 37*(4), 470–488.
4. van Hoof, J., Kort, H. S., Rutten, P. G., Duijnstee, M. S. (2011). Ageing-in-place with the use of ambient intelligence technology: Perspectives of older users. *International Journal of Medical Informatics, 80*(5), 310–31.

5. Demiris, G., Hensel, B. K., Skubic, M., Rantz, M. (2008b). Senior residents' perceived need of and preferences for "smart home" sensor technologies. *International Journal of Technology Assessment in Health Care, 24*(1), 120–124.
6. Bonato, P. (2010). Wearable sensors and systems. *IEEE Engineering in Medicine and Biology Magazine, 29*(3), 25–36.
7. Fatima, I., Fahim, M., Lee, Y. K., Lee, S. (2013). A unified framework for activity recognition-based behavior analysis and action prediction in smart homes. *Sensors, 13*(2), 2682–2699.
8. Hölscher, B. T. (2014). *The influence of obtrusiveness on the intention to advise the use of a wearable sensor of general practitioners*. Bachelor thesis, UVA.
9. Peek, S. T., Wouters, E. J., van Hoof, J., Luijkx, K. G., Boeije, H. R., Vrijhoef, H. J. (2014). Factors influencing acceptance of technology for aging in place: A systematic review. *International Journal of Medical Informatics, 83*(4), 235–248.
10. Cesta, A., Cortellessa, G., Giuliani, M. V., Pecora, F., Scopelliti, M., & Tiberio, L. (2007). Psychological implications of domestic assistive technology for the elderly. *Psychology Journal, 5*(3), 229–252.
11. Dautenhahn, K. (2007). Socially intelligent robots: Dimensions of human–robot interaction. *Philosophical Transactions of the Royal Society B: Biological Sciences, 362*(1480), 679–704.
12. Alami, R., Albu-Schäffer, A., Bicchi, A., Bischoff, R., Chatila, R., De Luca, A., et al. (2006). Safe and dependable physical human-robot interaction in anthropic domains: State of the art and challenges. In *IEEE/RSJ International Conference on Intelligent Robots and Systems,* October 9, 2006 (pp. 1–16). IEEE.
13. Rahimpour, M., et al. (2008). Patients' perceptions of a home telecare system. *International journal of medical informatics, 77*(7), 486–498.
14. Hirsch, T., Forlizzi, J., Hyder, E., Goetz, J., Kurtz, C., & Stroback, J. (2000). The ELDer project: Social, emotional, and environmental factors in the design of eldercare technologies. In *Proceedings on the 2000 Conference on Universal Usability* (pp. 72–79). ACM.
15. Giuliani, M. V., Scopelliti, M., & Fornara, F. (2005). Elderly people at home: technological help in everyday activities. In *IEEE International Workshop on Robot and Human Interactive Communication*. IEEE.
16. Ding, D., et al. (2011). Sensor technology for smart homes. *Maturitas, 69*(2), 131–136.
17. Mahoney, D. F., Purtilo, R. B., Webbe, F. M., Alwan, M., Bharucha, A. J., Adlam, T. D., et al. (2007). In-home monitoring of persons with dementia: Ethical guidelines for technology research and development. *Alzheimer's & Dementia, 3,* 217–226.
18. Steele, R., Lo, A., Secombe, C., & Wong, Y. K. (2009). Elderly persons' perception and acceptance of using wireless sensor networks to assist healthcare. *International Journal of Medical Informatics, 78*(12), 788–801.
19. Wu, Y. H., Damnée, S., Kerhervé, H., Ware, C., & Rigaud, A. S. (2015). Bridging the digital divide in older adults: A study from an initiative to inform older adults about new technologies. *Clinical Interventions in Aging, 10,* 193.
20. Mahoney, D. F., Mahoney, E. L., & Liss, E. (2009). AT EASE: Automated technology for elder assessment, safety, and environmental monitoring. *Gerontechnology, 8*(1), 11–25.
21. Scopelliti, M., Giuliani, M. V., & Fornara, F. (2005). Robots in a domestic setting: A psychological approach. *Universal Access in the Information Society, 4*(2), 146–155.
22. Warren, S. D., & Brandeis, L. D. (1890). The right to privacy. *Harvard Law Review, 15,* 193–220.
23. Westin, A. F. (1968). Privacy and freedom. *Washington and Lee Law Review, 25*(1), 166.
24. Schoeman, F. D. (Ed.), *Philosophical dimensions of privacy: An anthology*. Cambridge: Cambridge University Press.
25. Rochelandet, F. (2010). Économie des données personnelles et de la vie privée. *La Découverte*. July 1, 2010.
26. Zamani, K., Charalambidis, A., Konstantopoulos, S., Dagioglou, M., Karkaletsis, V. (2016). A peer-to-peer protocol and system architecture for privacy-preserving statistical analysis. In

International Conference on Availability, Reliability, and Security (pp. 236–250). Cham: Springer.

27. Coughlin, J. F., et al. (2007). Older adult perceptions of smart home technologies: Implications for research, policy & market innovations in healthcare. In *29th Annual International Conference of the IEEE Engineering in Medicine and Biology Society*. IEEE.
28. Mihailidis, A., Cockburn, A., Longley, C., & Boger, J. (2008). The acceptability of home monitoring technology among community-dwelling older adults and baby boomers. *Assistive Technology, 20*(1), 1–12.
29. Feil-Seifer, D., Matarić, M. J. (2009). Human robot interaction (HRI). In *Encyclopedia of complexity and systems science* (pp. 4643–4659). New York: Springer.
30. Riek, L., & Howard, D. (2014). A code of ethics for the human-robot interaction profession. In *Proceedings of We Robot*. Available at SSRN: https://ssrn.com/abstract=2757805.
31. Valkila, N., Litja, H., Aalto, L., & Saari, A. (2010). Consumer panel study on elderly people's wishes concerning services. *Archives of Gerontology and Geriatrics, 51*(3), e66–e71.
32. Boissy, P., Corriveau, H., Michaud, F., Labonte, D., & Royer, M. P. (2007). A qualitative study of in-home robotic telepresence for home care of community-living elderly subjects. *Journal of Telemedicine and Telecare, 13,* 79–84.
33. Demiris, G., et al. (2004). Older adults' attitudes towards and perceptions of 'smart home' technologies: A pilot study. *Medical Informatics and the Internet in Medicine, 29*(2), 87–94.
34. Demiris, G., Oliver, D. P., Dickey, G., Skubic, M., & Rantz, M. (2008). Findings from a participatory evaluation of a smart home application for older adults. *Technology and Health Care, 16*(2), 111–118.
35. Landau, R., Auslander, G. K., Werner, S., Shoval, N., & Heinik, J. (2010). Families' and professional caregivers' views of using advanced technology to track people with dementia. *Qualitative Health Research, 20,* 409–419.
36. Robinson, L., Hutchings, D., Corner, L., Beyer, F., Dickinson, H., Vanoli, A., Bond, A. (2006). A systematic literature review of the effectiveness of nonpharmacological interventions to prevent wandering in dementia and evaluation of the ethical implications and acceptability of their use. *Health Technology Assessment, 10,* iii, ix–108.
37. Sixsmith, A. J. (2000). An evaluation of an intelligent home monitoring system. *Journal of Telemedicine and Telecare, 6*(2), 63–72.
38. Stefanov, D. H., Bien, Z., & Bang, W. C. (2004). The smart house for older persons and persons with physical disabilities: Structure, technology arrangements, and perspectives. *IEEE Transactions on Neural Systems and Rehabilitation Engineering, 12*(2), 228–250.
39. Kang, H. G., et al. (2010). In situ monitoring of health in older adults: technologies and issues. *Journal of the American Geriatrics Society, 58*(8), 1579–1586.
40. Sharkey, A., & Sharkey, N. (2012). Granny and the robots: Ethical issues in robot care for the elderly. *Ethics and Information Technology, 14*(1), 27–40.
41. Blackman, T. (2013). Care robots for the supermarket shelf: a product gap in assistive technologies. *Ageing & Society, 33*(5), 763–81.
42. Smarr, C. A., Mitzner, T. L., Beer, J. M., Prakash, A., Chen, T. L., Kemp, C. C., Rogers, W. A. (2014). Domestic robots for older adults: attitudes, preferences, and potential. *International Journal of Social Robotics, 6*(2), 229–247.
43. Courtney, K. L., Demiris, G., & Hensel, Brian K. (2007). Obtrusiveness of information-based assistive technologies as perceived by older adults in residential care facilities: A secondary analysis. *Medical Informatics and the Internet in Medicine, 32*(3), 241–249.
44. Cesta, A., Cortellessa, G., Giuliani, V., Pecora, F., Rasconi, R., Scopelliti, M., & Tiberio, L. (2007a). Proactive assistive technology: An empirical study. In *IFIP Conference on Human-Computer Interaction* (pp. 255–268). Berlin Heidelberg: Springer.
45. Riek, L. D., Rabinowitch, T. C., Chakrabarti, B., Robinson, P. (2009). How anthropomorphism affects empathy toward robots. In *Proceedings of the 4th ACM/IEEE International Conference on Human Robot Interaction* (pp. 245–246). ACM.
46. Courtney, K. L., Demeris, G., Rantz, M., & Skubic, M. (2008). Needing smart home technologies: The perspectives of older adults in continuing care retirement communities.

47. Wild, K., Boise, L., Lundell, J., & Foucek, A. (2008). Unobtrusive in-home monitoring of cognitive and physical health: Reactions and perceptions of older adults. *Journal of Applied Gerontology, 27,* 181–200.
48. Gil, M., et al. (2013). Designing for user attention: A method for supporting unobtrusive routine tasks. *Science of Computer Programming, 78*(10), 1987–2008.
49. Demiris, G. (2009). Privacy and social implications of distinct sensing approaches to implementing smart homes for older adults. In *2009 Annual International Conference of the IEEE Engineering in Medicine and Biology Society* (pp. 4311–4314). IEEE.
50. Mynatt, E. D., et al. (2004). Aware technologies for aging in place: understanding user needs and attitudes. *IEEE Pervasive Computing, 3*(2), 36–41.
51. Chan, M., et al. (2009). Smart homes—Current features and future perspectives. *Maturitas, 64* (2), 90–97.
52. Reeder, B., Demiris, G., & Marek, K. D. (2013). Older adults' satisfaction with a medication dispensing device in home care. *Informatics for Health and Social Care, 38*(3), 211–222.
53. Zwijsen, S. A., Niemeijer, A. R., & Hertogh, C. M. P. M. (2011). Ethics of using assistive technology in the care for community-dwelling elderly people: An overview of the literature. *Aging & Mental Health, 15*(4), 419–427.
54. Townsend, D., Knoefel, F., & Goubran, R. (2011). Privacy versus autonomy: A tradeoff model for smart home monitoring technologies. In *Annual International Conference of the IEEE Engineering in Medicine and Biology Society*. IEEE.
55. Coeckelbergh, M. (2010). Health care, capabilities, and AI assistive technologies. *Ethical Theory and Moral Practice, 13*(2), 181–90.

Chapter 4
Realistic and Unobtrusive Solutions for Independent Ageing

M. Dagioglou, S. Ariño Blasco, D. Navarro Llobet and S. Konstantopoulos

4.1 Introduction

The purpose of the RADIO system is to support independent ageing by *providing assistance* to its primary users. At the same time, it *monitors* several *Activities of Daily Living (ADLs)* and collects clinically related information so that the clinical staff and/or informal caregivers (secondary users) can assess the level of independency of the elderly. The ultimate goal of the RADIO system is to provide its services to its primary and secondary users in an *unobtrusive way*.

As discussed in the previous chapter, obtrusiveness is a subjective, multidimensional, environment-dependent and multi-target[1] concept. In order to systematically and globally review the implications of obtrusiveness of the RADIO system, the dimensions proposed by Hensel et al. [1] were considered, namely: physical dimension, privacy, usability, function, human interaction, self-concept, routine and sustainability. The impact these dimensions have on the primary and secondary users depends on the requirements of each group.

Primary user requirements include all the requirements that the RADIO system must satisfy to offer a genuine improvement in elderly persons' quality of life. *Secondary user requirements* include: (a) the *clinical requirements* that is the

[1]RADIO system that is targeted to primary and secondary users. Moreover, an Ambient Assistive Living (AAL) environment can also impact people that do not live in it but spend time in it (e.g. visitors of the primary users, see Sect. 3.10 of Chap. 3).

M. Dagioglou (✉) · S. Konstantopoulos
Institute of Informatics and Telecommunications NCSR "Demokritos", Agia Paraskevi, Greece
e-mail: mdagiogl@iit.demokritos.gr

S. Ariño Blasco · D. Navarro Llobet
Fundació Privada Hospital Asil de Granollers, Granollers, Spain
e-mail: diananavarro@fhag.es

V. Karkaletsis et al. (eds.), *RADIO–Robots in Assisted Living*,
https://doi.org/10.1007/978-3-319-92330-7_4

clinical assessment items[2] to be monitored by the RADIO system and used by clinical staff to reliably recognize functional activity patterns and assess the independency of the primary user, and (b) the *caregivers' requirements* that prescribe the requirements that the RADIO system must satisfy to promote the caregivers' quality of life. Table 4.1 presents how the aforementioned requirements are contextualized within the obtrusiveness framework.

How we satisfy each requirement highly depends on the nature of each obtrusiveness dimension. Following, we group Hensel's dimensions of obtrusiveness in three macro-categories of constructs.

(a) ***Usability constructs***: usability and physical dimensions
(b) ***Utility constructs***: function and sustainability dimensions.
(c) ***Intrusiveness constructs***: privacy, human interaction, self-concept and routine dimensions.

Usability and utility constructs contain a high degree of objectivity and in that sense that they can be primarily controlled via: (a) technical requirements, design and evaluations and (b) piloting the system (user and medical evaluation).

On the other hand, the *intrusiveness construct* entails a high level of subjectivity that primarily depends on each primary user's perception and definition of all related concepts (privacy, human interaction, self-concept, dignity and routine). To this end, defining a universal framework that satisfies the needs of every potential user would be impossible. Satisfaction of these dimensions of obtrusiveness could be achieved, to a large extent, by obtaining individual consent and providing the option of selecting only the components that one does not find obtrusive. For example, a primary user could choose that the RADIO robot will not be equipped with visual sensors.

However, it is evident that this would completely undermine the utility of the system with respect to its clinical requirements. Thus, a clash is presented here between primary users' and clinical requirements, manifested primarily as *a gap between individual perceptions on privacy and, reliable and sound clinical information.*

In terms of privacy preservation, there are technical methods that can provide solutions to safeguard this. These solutions vary from how much information (content: raw data or descriptive statistics) is made available to interested parties (clinical staff, caregivers) to where the data are processed (on the sensors or in a central processing unit) and how these are managed. The content of information, particularly, plays a crucial role in clinical decision-making. From a clinical perspective, the technical solutions are required to provide sufficient information to allow for sound decisions.

Even though we cannot set a universal framework for satisfying obtrusiveness from the user's perspective, we can define for each monitored item *what is the most*

[2]In the RADIO system, InterRAI Long-Term Care Facilities and Home Care instruments were considered for selecting clinical requirementshttp://www.interrai.org/instruments/.

Table 4.1 Obtrusiveness dimensions and user requirements

Obtrusiveness dimension	User requirements (PU = primary users, SU = secondary users)
Physical	• Use of discrete, mobile and non-wearable sensors—*PU* • Control robot's proximity to user—*PU*
Usability	• Ease of interaction with RADIO: user-friendly GUIs—*PU* and *SU*
Privacy	• Privacy preserving data collection, management and access—*PU*
Function	• Reliable assistive services—*PU* • Reliable caregiver services (e.g. notifications)—*SU (caregivers)* • Reliable measurements and assessment items reporting—*SU (clinical items)*
Human interaction	• Facilitate communication with caregivers and social network—*PU* and *SU* • Being discrete so as not to discourage interaction with other people—*PU*
Self-concept	• Avoid stigmatizing symbols—*PU*
Routine	• RADIO system fulfills its medical purpose during user-initiated interactions. It does not interfere with daily activities solely for monitoring reasons—*PU*
Sustainability	• System designed to be affordable and extensible for future use cases—*PU* and *SU*

privacy preserving method that provides sufficient clinical information. Naturally, the balance between privacy preservation and sufficient clinical information is constrained by the state of the art of the technical methods.

In the following sections, we first discuss how the several aspects of the technical methods can become obtrusive in reference to primary users' and clinical requirements. We then go on with introducing a workflow that can be used as a guideline to extract the technical requirements for a system such as RADIO, and which bridges the gap between primary users' requirements and clinical requirements. These guidelines applied guarantee maximum unobtrusiveness for all involved parties.

4.2 Realistic Monitoring Solutions and Obtrusiveness Considerations

The methods for recognizing ADLs were introduced in Chap. 2. To study the extent to which each method can become obtrusive in reference to primary user and clinical requirements, one must consider: (a) the *sensors* used to collect *raw data* and (b) the subsequent *processing pipeline.*

The main question regarding the *source of data* collection is whether a sensing modality is obtrusive considering the specific activity or behaviour monitored as well as the area of a house where an item is monitored. It is thus evident that the sensors used to monitor primary users can collide with the requirements that result from *privacy considerations*. In the RADIO Home, data are collected by sensors that are either *fixed* or *mobile*. We discriminate *raw data collection* between four main sensing signals:

(a) *Audio data*, collected by microphones. These data are used for audio events recognition methods, identifying or verifying speakers, and non-verbal mood behaviour data. Moreover, audio data are used for automatic speech recognition.
(b) *Visual data*, collected by cameras. These data are used for human motion and posture analysis, face detection, recognition and expression analysis, as well as for clothes recognition for changing clothing detections.
(c) *3D/Range data*, collected by 3D cameras and laser scanners. Range data from a laser range finder are used to recognize motion patterns.
(d) *Smart Home data*, collected by Smart Home's automation and sensors. These data can provide some information about some ADLs such as locomotion by presence sensors as well as about electric appliances activity (power consumption) and bathing or toilet functions (water consumption).

In the processing pipeline that follows raw data collection, the main consideration is whether the ***type of information*** that comes as an output of each method is suitable to derive informed clinical decisions. In that sense, a method's outcome can collide with clinical requirements in terms of functional unobtrusiveness. The information collected for RADIO system can be presented into a hierarchy of increasingly privacy-respecting formats:

(a) *Raw content* that is the data collected by each sensor without any further processing,
(b) *Usage logs* that are a list of time-stamped activities and
(c) *Aggregates* on the usage logs.

Here we should note that especially for the visual sensors, there is an intermediate level between raw content and usage log, which deals with how visual data are represented, from pixelated representations to silhouette like ones (Chap. 2, Sect. 4.3).

The type of information needed to extract activity and behaviour information that satisfies clinical requirements depends on the nature of each clinical assessment item. Some items necessitate qualitative observations of 'how effortlessly somebody performed an activity'. In many such cases, this imposes disclosure of raw data as it is, except in the most trivial cases, impossible to automatically make such judgement. Other items are assessed on the basis of measurable quantities such as speed or occurrence frequency. Usage logs or aggregated types of information can provide such quantitative information. In some intermediate cases, a quantitative log can hint at qualitative information, although this is usually based on assumptions and premises that require careful consideration before we can safely assert the trustworthiness of this information.

Let us consider a hypothetical example where a visual sensor is used to observe the walking behaviour of a primary user. In this case, raw content is the actual video showing a person walking 4 m and could be used to assess any evidence of imbalance as this information is not available automatically. A detailed usage log would contain the performed speeds of several 4-m walk events within a day. Finally, aggregates of log can vary from descriptive statistics like an average of the day to more abstract information such as confirmation or not of an event.

With respect to the primary users, two major observations can be conducted regarding the type of information:

(1) A maximally privacy-respecting system would only provide aggregate information and, in fact, coarsely aggregated information (e.g. weekly Y/N).
(2) Human readable raw content presentation from audio and visual sensors, in the vast majority of activities and behaviour monitored, will be obtrusive to the primary users considering the privacy dimension.

To ensure respecting privacy, RADIO controls both the *collection* and the *processing* of raw content. Regarding the former, one of the system's main goals is to eliminate the necessity for wide coverage by multiple fixed cameras and to replace those with a single, mobile, visual sensor mounted on the robot. This is a compromise between the system's ability to safeguard safety and monitor relevant data and the end-users' sense of privacy: it is always easy to tell where the robot is looking and what is visible and what is not, it is always easy to not be in the same room as the robot, and at the same time the robot can proactively seek visual contact if necessary. In many important ways, a mobile visual sensor feels a lot closer to being cared after by a human companion than what the all-seeing eye of a wide-coverage CCTV installation feels like.

Regarding the transmission and processing of raw content, the following solutions can be used:

- Transmitting raw content to be processed at the RADIO Home's central processor. No raw content leaves the RADIO Home, however transmission over the RADIO Home wireless network does take place and raises security concerns. Raw content is not stored, but is deleted from the central processor's disk as soon as processing is completed. This allows maximal flexibility over the kinds of processing that can be performed.
- Attaching each sensor to each own lightweight processing unit. All image processing takes place in-memory immediately at the sensor. No raw visual content is stored or transmitted, not even within the RADIO Home network. Only abstract derivative information extracted from the raw data leaves the confines of the sensor. This, of course, comes with the downside on not being able to extract any more information from the raw data, other than the predefined features extracted.

In essence, *no raw content is available to any interested party*, in order to protect primary users' privacy. This naturally creates the following question: *What if raw content is needed to assess an item?* Here, a gap is created between primary user and medical requirements. In terms of technical solutions, the question is *if there is a solution (sensor and processing method) that provides to clinical staff the necessary information (functional unobtrusiveness) while protecting primary user's sensitive information (privacy unobtrusiveness).*

With this in mind, we go on to describe the process that we followed in RADIO in order to decide which items can be monitored.

4.3 Application of the Balancing Guidelines Methodology

The RADIO system's balancing guidelines include the methodology that balances between the primary user's and clinical requirements in situations where monitoring requirements necessitate obtrusiveness. The clinical requirements are *based on interRAI Long Term Care Facilities (LTCF) and Home Care (HC) Assessment systems* that consist of a list of items used by clinical staff to conduct a comprehensive assessment of the level of independency of elderly persons.

For each of these items, we consider:

1. *The monitoring sensors and methods* that can be used to collect relative information.
2. *The related primary user requirements* that are the obtrusiveness and ethical implications related to each item. For example, the use of visual sensors creates privacy concerns in self-performance activities such a dressing, toilet use bed mobility and it also creates human interaction and routine concerns in activities that involve others, such as eating.
3. *The type of information needed to satisfy the clinical requirements.* This is the type of information needed to extract medically informative content. For example, for all mood items, it is important that the number of times the behaviour is present (e.g. daily, present only once in the last 3 days, etc.) In 'bathroom usage', qualitative information is needed which cannot be safely inferred from quantitative information such as the mean number of bathroom usage events (usage log).

Figure 4.1 summarizes the workflow that can be followed to reach a decision for including or not an assessment item in the RADIO monitoring system. As a general rule: *an assessment item that raises obtrusiveness concerns can only be monitored if proper clinical assessment can be conducted based on usage logs or on aggregates on the logs.*

From the perspective of taking system architecture decisions following the balancing workflow, we can classify each method in three distinct *categories*:

1. Items where it is unclear how their recognition can be achieved, as it involves extracting qualitative information that is beyond the state of the art and would need novel algorithmic design. The only viable means is providing raw audiovisual content for observation by human caregivers, should this be acceptable by the primary users.

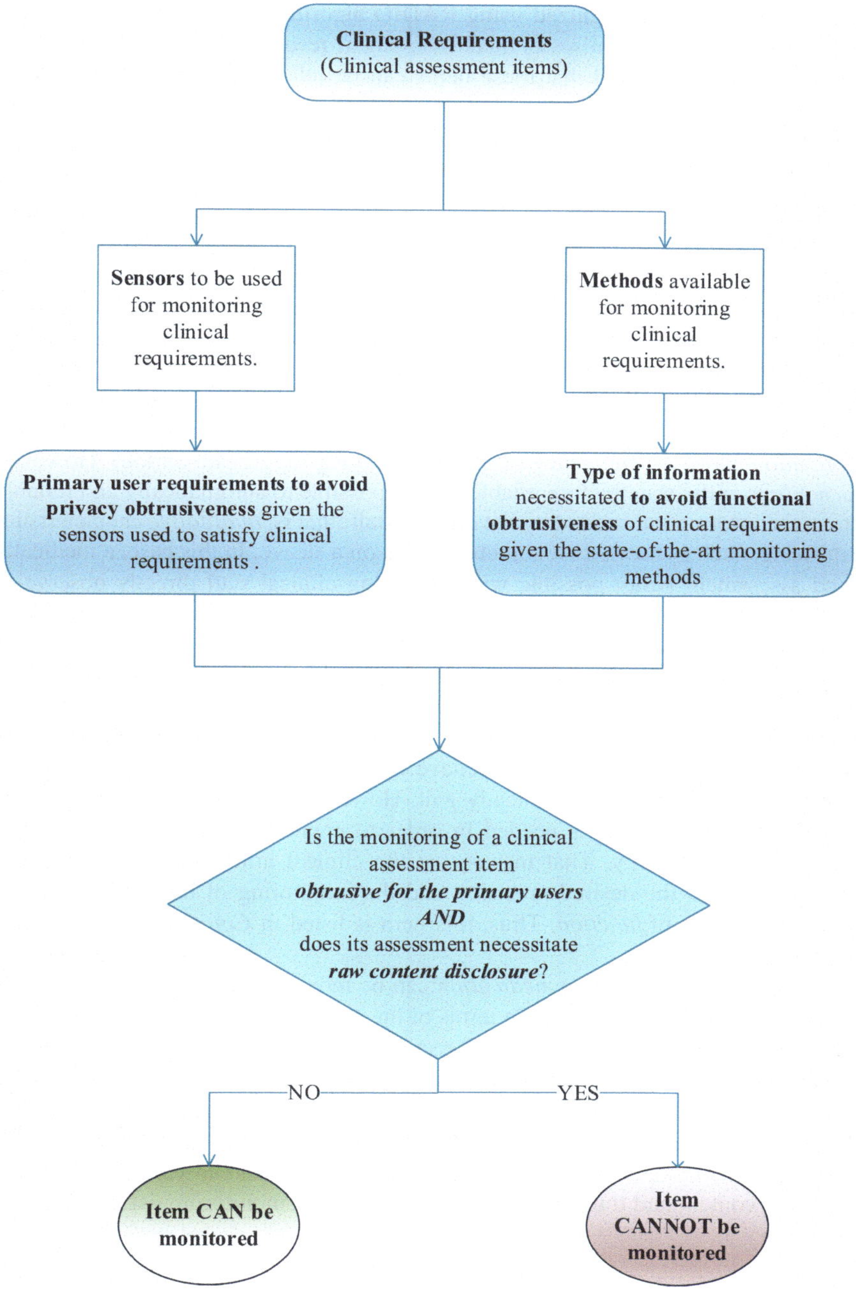

Fig. 4.1 Decision-making process for including an assessment item in a monitoring system. The final decision is a function of monitoring sensor and method used, the obtrusiveness dimensions related to each item and the information needed for medically sound decisions

2. Items that can be recognized using RADIO algorithms and methods, but at an accuracy that compromises clinical assessment results and functional unobtrusiveness. It is expected that these items can be reliably recognized in the near future, if they become the focus of engineering research effort.
3. Items that can be recognized using RADIO algorithms and methods at an acceptable accuracy and are included in the RADIO architecture.

Following we present three characteristic paradigms of how the aforementioned methodology was used.

The ADL self-performance item *Dressing upper body* can be monitored by *visual sensors*. This is potentially obtrusive in terms of the privacy dimension of obtrusiveness as it raises intimacy issues related to visual recordings. So, based on the decision tree in Fig. 4.1, monitoring the Dressing upper body item is *obtrusive* for the primary users. We then consider what is the least obtrusive information that can be provided. Using visual sensors, it is technologically possible to provide information about the frequency of clothes changing (aggregate on log). However, it is not (currently or in the foreseeable future) possible to automatically and reliably extract the information needed by the clinical staff; that is, *qualitative* characteristics of dressing, such as how *easily* somebody puts on a sleeve. In this case, a medically sound assessment is not possible without having clinical staff directly observe or watch recordings of (almost) raw visual content. Thus, this item is excluded from the list of monitored items as it belongs in *Category 1*.

The health condition item *Unsteady gait* is possible to be monitored by applying human walking pattern recognition methods on *range data*. Given the sensor used (laser scanner), this item is *not considered obtrusive* towards the primary users. There is no fundamental reason to believe that current pattern recognition cannot correctly and reliably assess unsteady gait. However, a major data collection and technical validation effort is needed in order to create the necessary models and establish their reliability. That means that the clinical information currently provided would lack the desired precision and the monitoring of this item would be *obtrusive* in terms of *function*. Thus, this item is listed in *Category 2* in the list of monitoring methods.

The iADL item *Managing medication* can be monitored by *visual sensors*. This item is also *potentially obtrusive* in terms of the privacy dimension of obtrusiveness due to intimacy issues related to visual recordings. So, again the monitoring of this item can be obtrusive for its primary users. Using visual sensors, it is technologically possible to provide information about pill intake occurrence (*usage log*). This information is useful for clinical staff who can thus detect impairment in this activity. In this case, a medically sound assessment is possible without disclosing raw visual content and thus this item is included in the monitoring list as it belongs in *Category 3*.

4.4 Further Considerations for Balancing Between Obtrusiveness and User Requirements

In the previous section, we presented a work flow that can be used to decide whether each clinical assessment item can be monitored unobtrusively for both primary and secondary users. However, in some cases, functional obtrusiveness is presented not solely on a one-item basis but on a group level. A characteristic example of such case is the monitoring of mood items. In this section, we discuss this phenomenon.

The standard Comprehensive Geriatric Assessment (CGA) process, both in the outpatient and institutional settings, involves the use of validated tools that help us to detect potential health problems. In the case of mood behaviour, the CGA performed through the interRAI LTCF or HC instruments considers 7 items: negative comments, persistent anger, unrealistic fears, health complaints, anxiety complaints, sadness-worries and crying. It is *the combination of these clinical variables that establishes the diagnosis of a problem.*

The precision of an assessment model tends to increase when independent predictors (assessment items) are added to the equation. It naturally follows that if we reduce these predictor variables, the power of the tool decreases. For example, the Yesavage geriatric depression scale originally consists of 30 items and has a cut-off point of 15 above which we suspect depression in the patient [2]. There are reduced versions of the Yesavage scale with 15 items and even versions of 10, 5, 4 items or 1 item [3, 4], but as we lower the number of variables we decrease sensitivity and specificity, decreasing thus the definitive clinical usefulness of the test. Scales with reduced items can potentially be used for early detection or screening, but not for strictly diagnostic purposes.

Obtaining information regarding affective state (negative comments, persistent anger, unrealistic fears, health complaints) through audiovisual sensors by means of interaction of the person with the robot (human–robot interaction HRI) by voice, speech, facial expression [5, 6] or by text analysis and doing so ‘unobtrusively’ is a great challenge.

State-of-the-art research related to emotional/mood detection reports accuracy percentages ranging between 50 and 60% [7]. Accuracy rates around 80% have been reported but these results are extracted on emotions deliberately pronounced in controlled environments and for particular sentences [8].

Therefore, based on current methods for detecting mood, reliable observations could not be guaranteed, rendering subsequent clinical usefulness uncertain. According to the Hensel model, this is related to the functional obtrusiveness dimension. Using a tool with such accuracy levels would impose decreasing the number of assessment items used. This would invalidate its reliability, validity, sensitivity and ultimately its clinical usefulness. It follows that if from the seven interRAI items we lose several due to detection methods immaturity/inaccuracy, the clinical usefulness is not as desired.

To sum up, in many occasions, the balancing guidelines must be complemented by ***a second-level analysis that involves considering functional obtrusiveness on a group level***. As discussed above, in some occasions, the reliability and usefulness of a behaviour assessment, such as mood, come as result of a group of items.

4.5 Tackling Overall Obtrusiveness

As explained earlier, the guidelines described above resolve the contradictions between primary users' and clinical requirements when these are contextualized within the obtrusiveness framework. In this way, we primarily guarantee unobtrusiveness in terms of privacy for the primary users and functional integrity for the

Table 4.2 Obtrusiveness dimensions and related RADIO actions

Obtrusiveness dimension	User requirements	RADIO actions
Physical	– Use of discrete, mobile, *not* wearable sensors – Control robot's proximity to user	– Overall system design – Technical work
Usability	– Ease of interaction with RADIO: user-friendly GUIs	– Usability pilot studies
Privacy	– Privacy preserving data collection, management and access	– Application of balancing requirements (as discussed above) – Home and ecosystem architecture design requirements and related technical work
Function	– Reliable assistive services for the PU – Reliable caregiver services (e.g. notifications) – Reliable measurements and assessment items reporting	– User evaluation during pilot studies – Caregivers' usability evaluation during pilot studies – Technical evaluation of methods and clinical evaluation of pilot studies
Human interaction	– Facilitate communication with caregivers and social network – Being discrete so as not to discourage interaction with other people	– Overall system design – Evaluation during pilot studies
Self-concept	– Avoid stigmatizing symbols	
Routine	– RADIO system fulfills its medical purpose during user-initiated interactions	
Sustainability	– System designed to be affordable and extensible for future use cases	– Evaluation of user's perspectives during pilot studies – Keeping bill of materials within reasonable for the target group budget – Sustainability, uptake and market positioning plan

purposes of clinical assessment. There are still several actions that must be taken in the design and development of system such as RADIO to ensure that overall unobtrusiveness is satisfied. These actions, that in many cases were hinted in Chap. 3, are summarized in Table 4.2 along with the user requirements.

4.6 Conclusions

One of the most challenging things that can be encountered while assigning obtrusiveness implications to a certain assessment item is the subjectivity of several constructs. For example, utility and usability constructs are somewhat objective and can be dealt with in the design, development and evaluation of the technical methods, as well as via the pilot studies during development of a system. However, intrusiveness constructs involve a highly subjective factor that boils down to each individual's preferences, ideology, cultural background, and viewpoint on health and dignity. Thus, universally establishing the ideal point of balance between obtrusiveness and medical requirements would be impossible.

What is possible, and has been achieved for the RADIO system, is to define the *framework* within which intrusiveness constructs should be discussed and negotiated. This framework elucidates the options that are technically feasible and clarifies each option's parameters and where these parameters stand with respect to both individual dignity and medical utility.

Naturally, many technological advances make this discussion more frictionless. The RADIO robot is one example, allowing monitoring that both has access everywhere if needed, but is not everywhere at all times. There are many more impressive examples, from blood sugar monitoring patches without sampling to modern surgical procedures, where the medical purpose is served better *and* in a less obtrusive way. What connects the examples above is the ability to easily explain how they differentiate themselves from their more obtrusive predecessors: a user can directly and immediately know what is being recorded, no blood sample is needed, recuperation time is shorter, etc.

For other technological advances, it might be hard to convincingly explain how they differ. The intrusiveness of extracting behavioural patterns from video content is a prime example. Most people will, perfectly understandably, connect being monitored by a visual sensor to disclosure of private moments in the form of video content. However, this is not necessarily true as the end product of data monitored via a visual sensor may only be a confirmation of the occurrence of an event or a statistical aggregation of event occurrences over longer of time. People who would not think twice about disclosing this latter, more abstract, information for medical reasons can (again, perfectly understandably) only reluctantly be convinced that a camera is not used to record video content but to extract abstract representations of behavioural indicators.

From a technical perspective, what is needed is the technical means to guarantee that video content cannot be extracted from such a device, and that this guarantee is a lot more absolute and convincing than what network security allows. RADIO pursued the development of visual sensors that directly extract abstract features without ever committing images to any computer memory (see Sect. 7.6 in Chap. 7), but non-technical work is also needed to create the mechanisms that can certify the correct operation of such non-recording visual sensors.

References

1. Hensel, B. K., Demiris, G., & Courtney, K. L. (2006). Defining obtrusiveness in home telehealth technologies: A conceptual framework. *Journal of the American Medical Informatics Association, 13*(4), 428–431.
2. Koehler, M., Rabinowitz, T., Hirdes, J., Stones, M., Carpenter, G. I., Fries, B. E., et al. (2005). Measuring depression in nursing home residents with the MDS and GDS: An observational psychometric study. *BMC Geriatrics, 5,* 1. Epub 2005/01/04.
3. Martinez de la, I. J., Onís-Vilches, M., Dueñas-herrero, R., Taberné-Aguado, C., Albert-Colomer, C. (2005). Abreviar lo breve. Aproximación a versiones ultracortas del cuestionario de Yesavage para el cribado de la depresión. *Aten Primaria, 35*(1).
4. Rinaldi, P., Mecocci, P., Benedetti, C., Ercolani, S., Bregnocchi, M., Menculini, G., et al. (2003). Validation of the five-item geriatric depression scale in elderly subjects in three different settings. *Journal of the American Geriatrics Society, 51*(5), 694–698.
5. Alonso-Martin, F., Malfaz, M., Sequeira, J., Gorostiza, J. F., & Salichs, M. A. (2013). A multimodal emotion detection system during human-robot interaction. *Sensors, 13*(11), 15549–15581.
6. Wang, K. C. (2015). Time-frequency feature representation using multi-resolution texture analysis and acoustic activity detector for real-life speech emotion recognition. *Sensors, 15*(1), 1458–1478.
7. Mano, L. Y., et al. (2016). Exploiting IoT technologies for enhancing health smart homes through patient identification and emotion recognition. *Computer Communications, 89,* 178–190.
8. Mao, Q., et al. (2014). Learning salient features for speech emotion recognition using convolutional neural networks. *IEEE Transactions on Multimedia, 16*(8), 2203–2213.

Part II
The RADIO System

Chapter 5
Integrating Robots and WSN: Communication and Interfacing Aspects

Christos P. Antonopoulos, Christos Panagiotou, Konstantinos Antonopoulos, Alexandros Spournias, Nikolaos Voros, Fynn Schwiegelshohn, Philipp Wehner, Michael Huebner, Diana Göhringer, Raquel Ventura, Alberto Fernández, Georgios Stavrinos and Evangelinos Mariatos

5.1 Conceptual RADIO Communication Architecture

5.1.1 End-to-End Conceptual Communication Architecture

The operating environments targeted by RADIO are domestic homes of elderly people. These homes, generally, do not have sufficient technological infrastructure

C. P. Antonopoulos (✉) · C. Panagiotou · K. Antonopoulos · A. Spournias · N. Voros
Embedded System Design and Application Lab, Computer and Informatics Engineering Department, Technological Educational Institution of Western Greece, Patras, Greece
e-mail: cantonopoulos@teiwest.gr

C. Panagiotou
e-mail: chpanag@teiwest.gr

K. Antonopoulos
e-mail: kostasantonop@cied.teiwest.gr

A. Spournias
e-mail: alexspou1@cied.teiwest.gr

N. Voros
e-mail: voros@teiwest.gr

F. Schwiegelshohn · P. Wehner · M. Huebner
Ruhr-University Bochum, Bochum, Germany
e-mail: fynn.schwiegelshohn@rub.de

P. Wehner
e-mail: philipp.wehner@rub.de

M. Huebner
e-mail: michael.huebner@rub.de

D. Göhringer
Technische Universitaet Dresden, Dresden, Germany
e-mail: diana.goehringer@tu-dresden.de

V. Karkaletsis et al. (eds.), *RADIO–Robots in Assisted Living*,
https://doi.org/10.1007/978-3-319-92330-7_5

to provide ad hoc ambient assisted living services. In order to guarantee that the impact of the RADIO system is not limited by requiring specific communication infrastructure to be prior deployed at the end-users' homes, the infrastructure connecting the RADIO components represents a substantial part of our architecture design. Specifically, the RADIO communication architecture includes: The wide-area communication between each RADIO Home and remote components, such as storage and processing facilities at the hospital or notification functionalities at care-givers' devices. The local, mostly (or even exclusively) wireless communication of the components deployed within each RADIO Home.

The RADIO Home environment itself comprises subgroups (Fig. 5.1), each fulfilling a different task and designed in response to different requirements

- Basic smart home: Off-the-shelf smart home devices
- Extended smart home: Advanced devices, integrating sensing and low-energy processing, as well as the RADIO Home server
- Mobile platform: Robotic platform, integrating sensors and limited computation functionality
- User interface devices.

In order to provide long-term support and reliability, the *basic smart home* sensor and actuator devices are off-the-shelf components such as Z-Wave products.

The *extended smart home subgroup* is based on Bluetooth to connect devices that carry out sensing and local processing in order to recognize daily activities and routines. This creates the requirement for a gateway that interfaces between Z-Wave and Bluetooth, in order to allow RADIO to combine the robustness offered by commercial Z-Wave devices with the flexibility to develop new services offered by Bluetooth.

Finally, the mobile platform establishes its own internal network in order to integrate its various sensing and processing elements, but also needs to connect to the overall RADIO Home. The platform is outfitted with two interfaces, the Bluetooth Low Energy (BLE) and the WiFi interface. BLE connectivity is provided

R. Ventura · A. Fernández
Sensing & Control Systems S.L., Barcelona, Spain
e-mail: raquel.ventura@sensingcontrol.com

A. Fernández
e-mail: alberto.fernandez@sensingcontrol.com

G. Stavrinos
Institute of Informatics and Telecommunications, NCSR "Demokritos", Agia Paraskevi, Greece
e-mail: gstavrinos@iit.demokritos.gr

E. Mariatos
AVN Innovative Technology Solutions, Limassol, Cyprus
e-mail: emariatos@avntechgroup.com

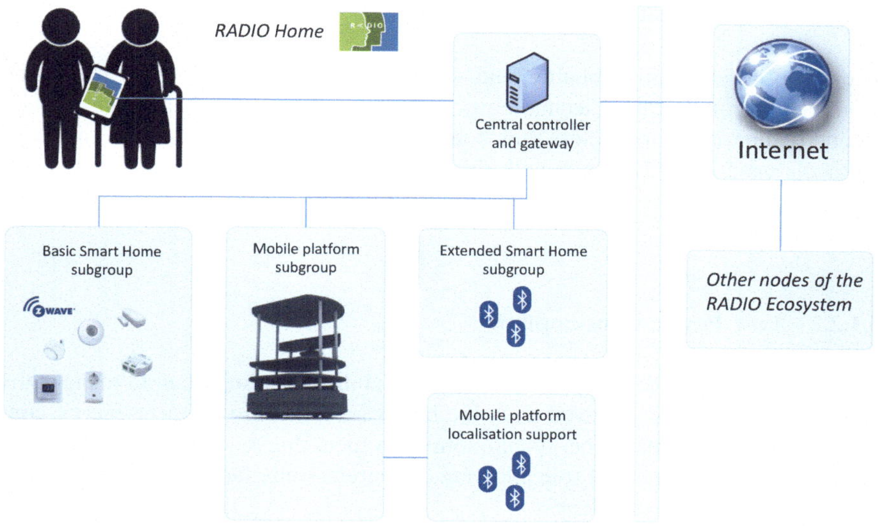

Fig. 5.1 Conceptual architecture of RADIO communication channels

to support direct access to devices of the extended smart home and WiFi connectivity for data transfer requirements.

This analysis gives us the architecture in Fig. 5.1 where the Z-Wave network, the Bluetooth network and the WiFi network interface at a *central gateway*. The gateway also serves as the central data processing point, since it is connected to all available devices in the smart home environment. Finally, the gateway interfaces with remote components of the RADIO ecosystem over the Internet.

5.1.2 Requirements at WSN Level

Wireless sensor networks, represent one of the fastest growing ICT sector, although posing stringent requirements, especially in the case where incorporated into an intelligent and assisted living environment, such as the ecosystem of the RADIO project [1]. The first important point aiming towards wide spread of a wireless sensors network, constitutes its design, so as to offer a useful and practical system for home environment monitoring. Also, especially in the case where installation takes place into user's private residence, it should offer high-level protection of personal data, as well as minimal obtrusiveness or discomfort to the user [2].

So, in this section, we analyze the requirements posed on wireless sensor network technologies, aiming to meet the objective of RADIO project. Such requirements take into account the end-users requirements in conjunction with the restrictions imposed by the existing technology of wireless sensor networks.

5.1.2.1 Communication Technology Support

The ability to efficiently, reliably, and securely transmit data wirelessly exploiting prominent communication technologies and protocols comprises the most fundamental requirement for wireless sensor network. This ability is related the variety of protocols used in RADIO and with different characteristics and requirements that each sensor may pose as well, thus drastically affecting complexity and energy consumption [2].

5.1.2.2 Low Power Consumption

Based on the assumption of scares energy availability, it is important to manage the node, both at software, as well as at the hardware level, to minimize energy consumption and to increase energy autonomy. To meet this requirement, MAC layer protocols play an important role allowing the wireless interface to enter low power mode during periods of idleness.

Another important factor drastically attributing to the overall WSN power consumption is the processing units of each sensor. Thus, in this aspect, wireless sensor manufacturers now offer several solutions, such as the well-known TI MSP430 and/or the ARM Cortex M family [1] yielding ultra-low power current demands and multiple low-power operational modes.

5.1.2.3 Data Throughput Capabilities

An important role in designing the wireless network pertains to the amount of data that can be efficiently transmitted during a specific time interval, which for the needs of RADIO project is low, so that it can easily be adapted to existing solutions. Towards such objectives multiple prominent ultra-low power communication technologies are explored (e.g., Z-Wave, IEEE 802.15.4, BLE, etc.) in order to optimally meet the data throughput requirements of the RADIO application scenarios.

5.1.2.4 Delay—Jitter Requirements

Another requirement to be met, has to do with the delay variance of the receiving data packets from sensors particularly considering data streams. In this case, packets are sent in a continuous stream evenly spaced. Due to network congestion, improper queuing, or configuration errors, this steady stream can become lumpy, or the delay between each packet can vary. Respective technologies used must make sure that predefined time deadline is not violated.

5.1.2.5 Easy and Rapid Connection Support

On connection's supporting side between two nodes, there are two techniques, which are the connection-based and the connectionless, with respectively advantages and disadvantages.

Connectionless communication, on the one hand uses low complex protocol such as IEEE 802.15.4, as there is no need for additional mechanisms to establish and/or terminate a connection. Also, such a communication makes it easier to create multi-hop and mesh networks. On the other hand, they do not offer inherent support to QoS, robust data transfer, load balancing and in general traffic control, something that is required to offer in nowadays WSNs, as their applications increase the criticality, complexity and communication requirements.

On the other side, considering connection-based linking of two nodes, there is usually a scenario, where a node is used as a master and the other node as a slave. This technique provides data traffic load anticipation, Quality of Service, which allows to prepare an effective packet transmission timing. This approach is traditionally followed by Bluetooth technology. Each approach offers specific advantages and disadvantages and correct selection is critical in order to meet end-user demands.

5.1.2.6 Security Support

As the popularity and expansion of WSNs are increasing, the support of data security becomes mandatory, especially when applied into demanding areas such as health care and welfare of users, as it relates directly to the management and distribution of sensitive personal data. In RADIO project, three services are used to support security.

The first service is data privacy, which ensures that data can be useful only on nodes that can understand that. The second service refers to the authentication of node, which ensures that it is authorized, to receive and/or send data. The last third service provides authorization as it determines the level of access that can have a particular user to certain data and/or functions and is inextricably linked to the authentication service.

5.1.3 Requirements at Backend Level

RADIO poses several requirements for its backend platform as they are introduced by the multifaceted nature of the services that RADIO offers. IoT technologies lead to a rapid increase of the data sources and respectively to a massive growth of the volume of modalities that demand data storage and processing. This is the context that the Big Data problem describes. Particularly, the IoT and Big Data challenges are identified by the three Vs [3]. **Three Vs** stand for **(1) Volume, (2) Velocity, and**

(3) Variety. **Volume**, as the term implies, refers to the excessive amount of data that an IoT platform needs to handle. **Velocity** describes the high speed of the data flow, change and processing. Finally, **Variety** defines all kind of diversity that is present in data, data models, query languages and data sources.

In a more fine-grained view, these three main classes of challenges, that are also present in the RADIO infrastructure backend level, can be broken-down in several other challenges that give more insights towards a modern IoT platform [4]:

Scalability: Scalability is not applied only in terms of the number of sensors and actuators connected to the system, or the networks that interconnect them. Rather scalability concerns the amount of data associated with the system and the data rate and the amount of processing power required. With the number of data sources integrated to an IoT system always increasing, the need for a scalable IoT Backend that scales efficiently is a major requirement that drives the architecture design of the backend.

Heterogeneous modalities: Modern IoT systems depend on the analysis of vast quantities of data. In order to extract patterns and meaningful information from high volumes of raw and heterogenous data (sensor readings, video footage, etc.) the need to efficiently support highly demanding processing tasks is required by the IoT backend platform. Such requirements can be addressed in pair with the need for scalability, through the adoption of microservices approach. Processing tasks can be identified as isolated microservices able to operate in a sandbox environment and scale efficiently when required.

Cloud computing: IoT backend systems involve the use of cloud computing platforms. Cloud computing platforms increased the availability of storage and processing resources and through the microservices approach achieve even more efficient utilization of these resources. Cloud computing and microservices are the two technologies that lead to the development of flexible and scalable cloud services and the efficient integration with IoT systems. RADIO backend comprises by two distinct IoT platforms, thus being highly adaptable and able to deal with new requirements, firmware or system updates and offer new capabilities over time.

Real time: IoT systems often operates in application domains where real time is required. Streams of data are continually transferred to the backend system which must respond in predefined time windows. The real-time requirements concern, processing of the data stream, decision making based on the events produced and final reaction. In most time critical application domains, where real time is required, the result of violating the real time constraints could lead in catastrophic results for assets, infrastructures or even human life.

Highly distributed: IoT systems can span large geographical areas. In that sense, data can be stored at the edge of the network or stored centrally in the backend platform. While processing can take place at the edge of the network, either in the IoT gateways or even in sensors and actuators the most critical and intensive tasks takes place centrally in backend infrastructure and offered as cloud services. Despite the high level of distribution, IoT Backend platforms are a fundamental component of an IoT ecosystem that are responsible at least for persisting the state of the system and harmonizing raw data and extracted information.

RADIO backend platform is the center of the RADIO system that guarantees the data storage, processing and service delivery for all involved end-users.

Security and Privacy: The mass adoption of IoT devices in various sectors of social and economic life that vary from personal residences to industry and health premises demand security and privacy concerns to be addressed convincingly. Regardless the application domain and its functional requirements, security and privacy of IoT systems is a requirement that is always present and thus, given solutions must scale and evolve with the systems. Security and privacy in RADIO is addressed through encrypted communication through adequate APIs, strong authentication and authorization mechanisms and encrypted data storage.

Compliance and Standardization: The wide variety of data sources and technologies have already lead to a fragmentation that make the need for standardization in IoT a challenge of major importance. Moreover, since these systems, as already noted, are applied in demanding environments must comply with rules and regulations that provide the appropriate confidence to the stakeholders of the IoT systems. Thus, RADIO APIs comply with adequate standard communication models.

Integration Capabilities: IoT evolution was driven by the need for delivering communication of physical devices (things) that are uniquely identified in a common network (Internet) and interact with other devices, services and end-users. Therefore, the requirement for seamless integration for devices applied in various domains (home appliances, wearables, automation and control systems, online services, etc.) is highlighted as the cornerstone for IoT Platforms. In that respect, the RADIO backend platform communicates with the rest of the RADIO ecosystem (sensors, actuators, robot, gateways) through a homogeneous way offering both HTTP as well as MQTT messaging protocol support.

5.2 Integrated Wireless Communication Technologies and Bridging Considerations

5.2.1 Introduction to Z-Wave and Interfaces

Z-Wave is one of the communication protocols used within connected world to exchange information between smart products. A communication protocol defines how signals are sent from one device to another. Z-Wave operates at the low frequency 918/960 MHz band, meaning interference is minimal. Z-Wave uses AES-128 symmetric encryption for security. There are a wide range of devices compatible with Z-Wave, around 2400 supported devices and 700 members associated. Some smart home brands and devices that support Z-Wave include: Samsung SmartThings, Wink hub, Honeywell thermostats, Hogar Milo, Somfy, LG SmartThiq.

Z-Wave devices use a proprietary protocol from Sigma Designs, http://www.sigmadesigns.com. Respective devices can communicate directly, but in the most common case, they form a wireless network being managed by a node called controller. The controller is responsible to manage the Z-Wave network and Z-Wave devices, while APIs are provided to the controller application in order to create simple or complex systems through the combination of the different device functionalities that forms the network. In the case of Sensing & Control's smart home system, the system provides functions for security, comfort, home automation and energy management.

Figure 5.2 shows the chosen hardware device that brings Z-Wave connectivity in order to communicate with Z-Wave products. The controller (gateway) and smart home application use the Z-Wave module called RaZberry for the Raspberry Pi.

In the smart home, the Z-Wave gateway is the only point for communication between Z-Wave devices and the corresponding remote elements of the RADIO ecosystem, i.e., the respective IoT Platform.

In the first integrated prototype, the clients of the Z-Wave Smart Home devices needed to access devices through the RESTful API provided by the cloud-based IoT Platform. In the last prototype, the RADIO Home Controller was capable of communicating smart home devices with external services without using the cloud-based IoT platform. A fully local RESTful API was implemented that allows client functions to access data structures in Z-Wave and execute per devices and handling network management functions. This allows client functions to be integrated within the smart home application by running in the local controller.

Client functions integrated within the smart home application running in the Z-Wave gateway can result in high computational cost depending on the complexity of the client functions and the gateway's limited hardware resources (CPU and RAM memory). Therefore, this architecture requires a priori evaluation in order not to reduce the performance of the smart home functions already implemented into the gateway.

The local RESTful API implements the whole control logic of the Z-Wave network. The two main functions are

- Management of the network. This includes adding and removing devices and managing the routing of the network. In the Z-Wave terminology all these functions are called 'function classes'. They are functions offered by the controller itself.
- Execution of commands through "command classes" that allows the control of Z-Wave device functions. Command classes offer the variables and the commands according to the abilities of the respective devices. Command classes consist of two types of commands: commands for users (most of them are "GET" and "SET") and commands for configuration.

Most of the Z-Wave commands can be controlled by the local RESTful API but only a small subset is accessible for external applications for security reasons.

The basic Z-Wave commands accessible for external applications are

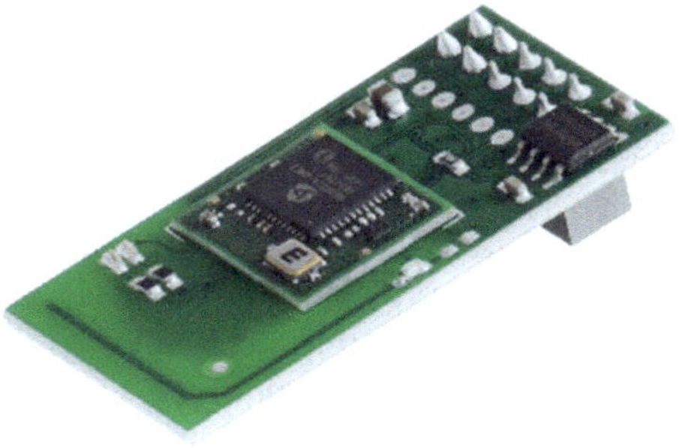

Fig. 5.2 z-Wave module (called RaZberry) for interfacing the gateways to the Z-Wave network

Z-Wave command	Type of class
sendData	FUNCTION_CLASS
AddNodetoNetwork	FUNCTION_CLASS
RemoveNodeFromNetwork	FUNCTION_CLASS
setValue	FUNCTION_CLASS
SetNodeLocation	FUNCTION_CLASS
SetNodeName	FUNCTION_CLASS
toggleActuatorSensor	COMMAND_CLASS
toggleDimmableSensor	COMMAND_CLASS
setThermostatSetPoint	COMMAND_CLASS
setThermostatMode	COMMAND_CLASS
setThermostatFanMode	COMMAND_CLASS

5.2.2 Introduction to BLE and Interfaces

Bluetooth is a wireless radio specification designed to replace cables as the medium for data and voice signals between electronic devices. The specification is defined by the Bluetooth Special Interest Group (SIG) which is made up of over 1000 electronics manufacturers. Intended primarily for mobile devices, Bluetooth's design places a high priority on small size, low power consumption and low costs. The Bluetooth specification seeks to simplify communication between electronic devices by automating the connection process.

Bluetooth radios operate in the unlicensed 2.4 GHz Industrial, Scientific, and Medical application (ISM) frequency range. Since this frequency is already widely used by other devices, to avoid interference from these devices, Bluetooth uses a technology called spread spectrum frequency hopping. Spread spectrum frequency hopping changes the transmission frequency up to 1600 times per second across 79 different frequencies. As a result, interference on any one of those frequencies will only last a fraction of a second. This, coupled with the limited range of Bluetooth radio transmitters, results in a robust signal that is highly tolerant of interfering devices sharing the same frequency.

Bluetooth-based solutions' performance can vary significantly depending both on the version of the protocol supported and even more on the specific implementation's characteristics. Therefore, concerning data rates solutions covering a wide range from 300 Kbps up to 1.5 Mbps can be found. Indicative examples of relative solutions include Shimmer [5] and MoviSens [6] platforms. The former is utilized in the Roving Networks based Bluetooth modules [7].

The latest version of the standard, Bluetooth Low Energy (BLE), represents a different technology from Classic Bluetooth (and in fact incompatible technology) being promoted by the Bluetooth Special Interest Group (SIG) and benefitting of the hugely successful Classic Bluetooth it shows significant dynamics compared to analogous technologies being incorporated. Furthermore, it offers high degree of flexibility both concerning implementation approaches and communication approaches supporting different ways for nodes to communicate through different data structure profiles to best fit the application requirements. Both these aspects were critical for the RADIO objectives highlighting relative solutions as good candidates for RADIO purposes. The main fundamental step was to actually evaluate respective solutions and realistically verify that the performance offered is adequate for the goals of the project.

The increased adoption of the BLE technologies in the IoT domain has enabled researchers, companies and the Bluetooth Special Interest Group (SIG) to explore the feasibility of mesh networking over BLE. Currently, enhancements focused on mesh networking are on the roadmap of all the BLE related vendors. BLE mesh support is expected to provide new capabilities and increase the IoT functionalities.

Dominant players in the market of low power wireless SoCs and BLE particularly have already released their first efforts towards mesh enabled BLE networks. Since the standardization of a mesh mechanism for BLE has not been finalized yet, each company is working on its own version of mesh networking over Bluetooth [8–11].

5.2.3 Introduction to ZigBEE and Interfaces

ZigBee is an open standard wireless protocol, build on top of IEEE 802.15.4, developed by ZigBee Alliance. ZigBee is particularly targeted at low-power, low-cost and low data rate wireless sensors and control networks. Aimed at interoperability, it emphasizes on low complexity implementation and can support connectivity of up to 65,000 nodes. ZigBee operates at three different frequency bands including 868, 915 MHz and 2.4 GHz. Using the most popular frequency band, at 2.4 GHz, ZigBee nodes can communicate within a distance of up to 100 m, with a maximum throughput of 250 Kbps.

A ZigBee node that performs all the tasks defined by ZigBee standard is called a Full-Function Device (FFD). In contrast to an FFD, a Reduce-Function Device

(RFD) is a ZigBee node with limited tasks, which can only connect to an FFD. With respect to these functionalities, ZigBee devices can be classified in three types, namely Coordinator, Router and End Devices. A ZigBee Coordinator is a Full-Function Device, and a ZigBee network can contain only one. Its main responsibilities are the initial setup of the ZigBee network as well as the overall management of it. Main functions of the ZigBee Coordinator include address allocation, granting permission to nodes to join or leave the network and transfer application data. Due to the criticality of this node on a ZigBee network, it must always be powered on. A ZigBee Router is another Full-Function Device. A ZigBee network can contain none, one or more routers, depending on the size and the topology of the network. Its main functionality is to expand a ZigBee network. More specifically, it performs all the functions of the ZigBee Coordinator except network establishment. Constant power source must also be provided for a ZigBee Router.

A ZigBee End Device is a Reduce-Function Device, which located at the edges of a network. Its main functionality is to transmit and receive data. In order to conserve resources, ZigBee End Devices turn off their radio when they are idle and this where ZigBee as wireless communication technology emphasizes on power conservation.

5.2.4 Bridging WSN and WiFi Interfaces in RADIO

The smart home is comprised of several devices with different communication protocols. Figure 5.3 shows all available devices within the smart home environment and their respective interconnections. The RADIO Robot is presented in more detail in Chap. 6 of this volume, but what is relevant to the discussion here is that the robot's software is integrated using the Robot OS (ROS) middleware, with WiFi used to physically connect ROS nodes executing on the robot with ROS nodes executing on an off-board Raspberry Pi. This off-board unit also integrates the ROS WiFi network with the Z-Wave network and the BLE network as follows:

- One module is simultaneously a node of the ROS middleware and a node of the MQTT middleware used by the BLE network, and copies messages between the two.
- One module is simultaneously a node of the ROS middleware and a client of the REST API to the Z-Wave network provided by the Z-Wave Gateway, and copies messages between the two.

It should be noted that there is no direct bridge between the two WSN networks. Such a bridge is not needed, as both sensor networks only need to communicate with the Main Controller (see Sect. 3.1)*, which is main information broker of the overall system.

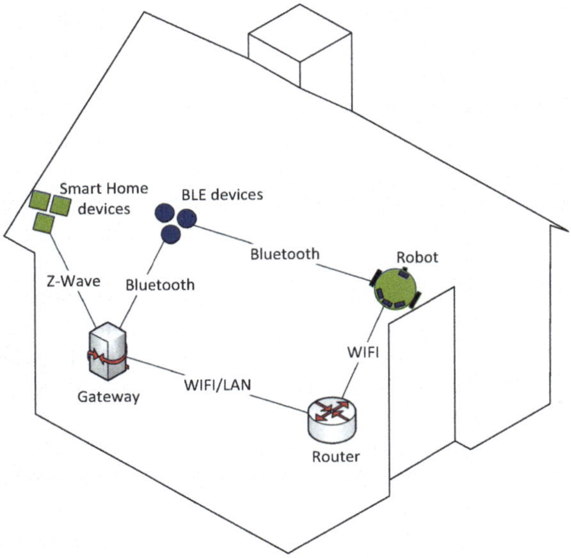

Fig. 5.3 Device interconnection within the smart home environment

Since the robot should act autonomously and not be controlled remotely, it needs to be interconnected to the smart home environment. The robot is outfitted with two processing platforms: an Intel NUC and an Avnet PicoZed. The NUC is responsible for controlling the base platforms sensors and actuators. Therefore, it is directly connected to the TurtleBot2 base platform via USB. The Avnet PicoZed serves as accelerator platform to reduce the computation load of the Intel NUC. Additional devices that are placed on the robot are an Asus Xtion Pro camera and a Hokuyo laser scanner. These two devices can either be connected to the Intel NUC or to the Avnet PicoZed. The Intel NUC supports two wireless communication interfaces, the Bluetooth Low energy (BLE) and the WIFI interface. BLE connectivity is used for localization tasks performed by the robot, while the WIFI interface is required to connect the smart home environment to the IoT platform.

Initial measurements have shown that the usage the BLE and WIFI transceiver simultaneously results in degraded RSSI performance of the BLE transceiver. This is because the localization task requires accurate readings of the received signal strength indication values of the respective BLE devices. Because both interfaces are placed on the same network chip, the WIFI interface interferes with the BLE interface and vice versa. Additionally, both signals use the ISM band around 2.4 GHz so that spectral overlapping of the signals can occur. This can results in strong signal interference. Exemplary measurements are shown in Figs. 5.4 and 5.5.

The figures show the signal strength in dBm over the frequency in GHz. The left spectrum of Fig. 5.4 depicts the spectrum of the BLE broadcaster. The three peaks show the frequency band of an advertising channel of the spectrum. They are highlighted in yellow. The mean value of the signal strength equals to −41.3 dBm. In contrast, the right spectrum of Fig. 5.4 shows the spectrum over 2.4 GHz

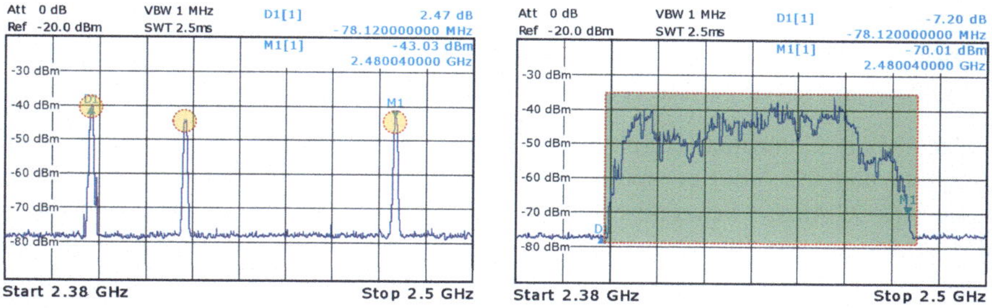

Fig. 5.4 Spectrum BLE (left) and 2.4 GHz WIFI (right)

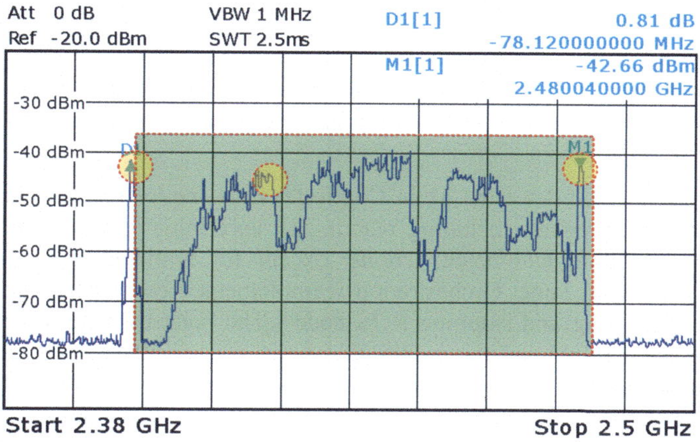

Fig. 5.5 Spectrum BLE and WIFI

802.11 b/g/n wireless LAN transceiver. Its region of influence starts at 2.395 GHz and ends at 2.484 GHz and is highlighted in green. The mean signal strength equals to approximately −44 dBm. The combination of both signals is shown in Fig. 5.5. Based on the measurements shown in the spectrums in Fig. 5.4, an overlapping of the signals can be seen in the frequency band. Especially the advertising channel 38 is located in the WIFI spectrum. In order to reduce this interference, an external WIFI USB interface is used and connected to the Intel NUC.

5.3 RADIO Gateway Component

5.3.1 Main Controller

The RADIO Main Controller is the main orchestrator of the behaviours of the RADIO Home and the main keeper of the information collected and analyzed by the various RADIO Home systems. Its functionalities include

- System orchestration
- Bridging between the different subsystems
- Storing and serving ADL recognition results.

The Main Controller is (physically) partially distributed between the home computer and the robot computer, via a multi-master architecture: the core ROS process (*ROS Master*) executes on both the robot's on-board computer and on an off-board Raspberry Pi and messages are copying between the two integrate the two subsystems. This adds integration complexity compared to having ROS nodes (possibly remotely) connect to a single ROS Master, but it resolves the deadlock that

- Many RADIO Home functionalities do not depend on the robot. If a single ROS Master executes on the robot, the Main Controller would be unable to operate with the robot turned off or having run out of battery.
- If a single ROS Master executes off the robot, the bandwidth-hungry communication channels between the sensors and the perception modules would have to use the Wifi.

An important module of the Main Controller if the *node manager* that orchestrates the overall system, including reacting to user initiatives through the user device and initiating automated actions, except for home automation directly handled by the S&C suite. Orchestration is implemented by sending control messages and by starting and stopping ROS nodes. The node manager also monitors ROS node execution to restart nodes that have crashed. The node manager is distributed between the on-board and the off-board computer and is implemented as two ROS nodes. The main node is the one executing on the off-board computer, and it relegates to the on-board node the distribution of control messages for the system components that execute on the robot. Only the main node is required for the operation of the overall RADIO Home, so that functionalities not related to the robot remain active even if the robot is off-line or turned off.

5.3.2 Z-Wave GW

The Z-Wave gateway is responsible to manage the Z-Wave network and Z-Wave devices, while providing APIs to the controller application in order to create simple or complex systems through the combination of the different device functionalities that forms the network. The Z-Wave gateway initiates control commands and sends out the commands to devices and IoT platform. The controller has the capability to include/exclude nodes in the network and therefore always have the latest network topology. The controller device has a full routing table and is therefore able to communicate with all nodes in the Z-Wave network. The routing table is where the controller keeps the information from the nodes about the network topology. The routing table is built by the controller based on information received from all the nodes in the network, at installation time, about each nodes range.

In the case of Sensing & Control's smart home system, the system provides functions for security, comfort, home automation and energy management. The Z-Wave gateway provides three important functions

(1) Management of Z-WAVE network and devices
(2) Basic preprocessing capabilities (mainly energy calculations)
(3) Local information repository in order to deal with temporal Internet cut offs (so Historical information is stored and sent when Internet connectivity is resumed).

In addition, the gateway has both computational resources and physical interfaces that can be used to connect third-party transceivers to enable connectivity via other communication protocols, such as WiFi or Bluetooth. The controller is composed by (i) a logical division of Java code named as Hardware Abstraction Layer (HAL) that bridges the gap between different hardware architectures and software by providing a uniform interface to the system peripherals, and (ii) a set of Java programs that provide different features, including a rules engine for setting "if this, then that" style rules for how things interact (Fig. 5.6) and a scheduler for enabling to set up the time that an action will be executed (Fig. 5.7). For instance, you can trigger an action at a specific time (an hour of the day) or during a specific period (day, night or other intervals of time), and on given days. The user can also schedule an action to repeat itself several times.

Additional functions may also be integrated to run on the gateway if their resource consumption (or computational cost) is equal or less a predefined acceptable level, i.e., without compromising the overall performance of the RADIO solution. The growing number of IoT devices and dependency between them require a faster and smarter approach than the traditional one (gathering data and sending them through networks to the cloud to be processed). Fog computing architecture pushes the intelligence and processing power to the local area network level through the gateway. For RADIO, the gateway was delivered running on Raspberry Pi and Linux-enabled.

5.3.3 BLE GW

In this section the presented gateway, shown in Fig. 5.8 aggregating data transmitted over Bluetooth Low Energy (BLE) wireless technology, but not limited only to BLE, in the context of the RADIO.

The high-level design, of the Gateway architecture consists from three main components, namely the Kernel, Applications and the Messaging Bus. At the lower layer of the architecture lies the Kernel of the Gateway, where the core modules are deployed. On the contrary, at the top of the architecture, user-defined applications

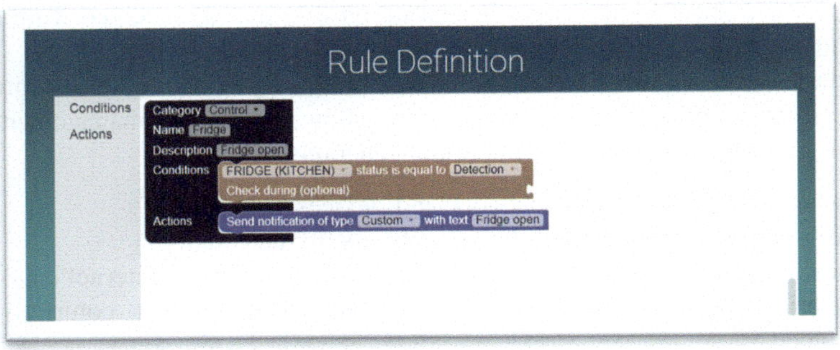

Fig. 5.6 Setting a rule to receive a customized notification

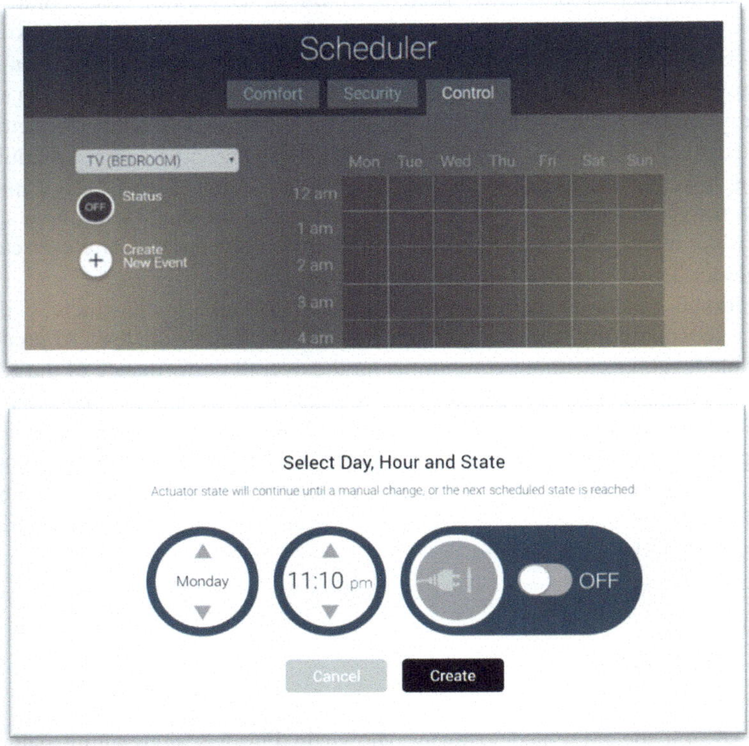

Fig. 5.7 Scheduling an action on the TV device

are commissioned, typically requiring a considerably higher degree of flexibility. Finally, in order to assure efficient interconnection between the two aforementioned components, a dedicated intermediate layer, the Messaging Bus, is introduced providing intra Gateway communication capabilities and functionalities.

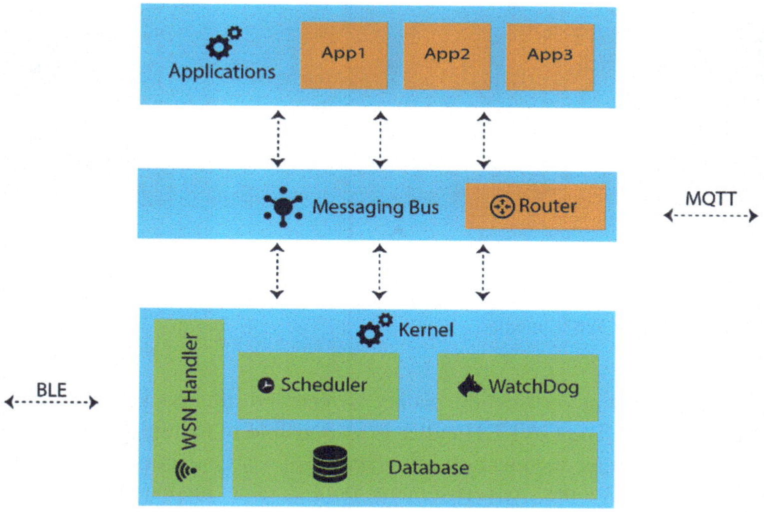

Fig. 5.8 BLE gateway high-level architecture

BLE Gateway Kernel

The WSN Handler, shown in Fig. 5.9, is the main aggregation point for operations associated with the Wireless Sensor Networks, and more specifically with BLE networks. Due to the fact that the communication between devices, in a BLE network, can be either connection-oriented or connectionless, the WSN Handler divided in three submodules, namely Advertisements Publisher, Advertisements Scanner and GATT Handler. The Advertisements Publisher and Scanner are handling the connectionless communication, where GATT Handler handle the connection-oriented communication.

The main entry point for the BLE advertisement packets is the Advertisements Scanner, where every advertisement packet received on the BLE interface, is being considered. Next, according to the advertisement type, exported by the BLE PDU, the received packet forwarded to the appropriate module or discarded. There are many types of advertisement packets according to the Bluetooth Specification [12]. In the case of RADIO platform, Advertisements Scanner identifies solely the two following types of advertisements:

1. ADV_NONCONN_IND, Non-connectable undirected advertising. Used by devices that want to broadcast and don't want to be connected or scannable. This is the only option for a device that is only a transmitter.
2. ADV_DIRECT_IND, Connectable directed advertising. Directed advertising is used when a device needs to connect to another device.

When an *ADV_NONCONN_IND* advertisement packet received, the Advertisement Scanner forwards it to all interested parties. In contrast, when an

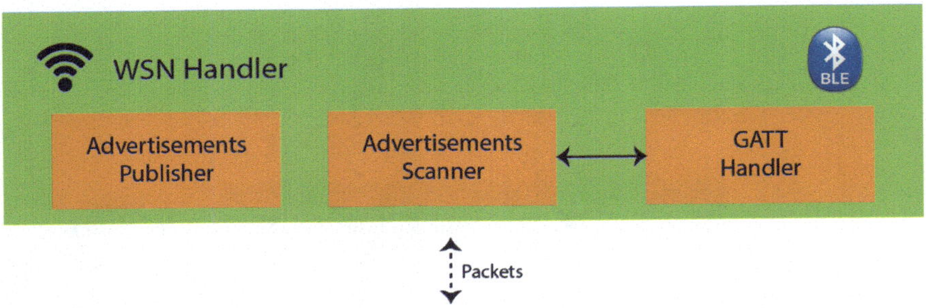

Fig. 5.9 BLE gateway WSN handler

ADV_DIRECT_IND advertisement packet is received, this packet is forwarded to the GATT Handler. The GATT Handler is responsible to handle all the lifecycle of a BLE Device, such as, Connection initialization, Data Collection, and Connection Termination. Finally, the Advertisement Publisher is responsible to broadcast messages originated from the Gateway to the BLE network.

Database module, as the name implies, provides data persistence capabilities in the gateway. The Scheduler module, is a dynamic scheduling mechanism exposing functionalities for other modules and applications to execute simple or long running tasks.

Watchdog component is the main monitoring tool of the Gateway. It monitors all hardware and software components of the Gateway and periodically sends respective data and system metrics to the Backend infrastructure. In this way administrators can effectively maintain the overall status of the deployed gateways.

Messaging Bus

The Messaging Bus is the main aggregation point for all incoming and outgoing messages related to the Gateway. Internally, it offers local MQTT connections among the Gateway modules and applications. Externally, it maintains MQTT connections to the respective IoT Backend infrastructure, in order for the Gateway to communicate with IP networks. Due to the existence of two different messaging systems, the internal Gateway messaging system (Modules, applications communication), and the external messaging system (Backend IoT infrastructure communication), the need for a module was raised to bridge these two systems. To tackle this need, the Router plugin is added to the design, inside the Messaging Bus. The plugin performs topic-based routing by intercepting messages from topics, analyzing them and finally forwarding them, to the appropriate, external or internal MQTT topics, without modifying the message content.

User-Defined Applications

At the top level of the architecture, the Applications component, is responsible to dynamically deploy and manage all user-defined applications that run on the gateway. Applications resides outside the Gateway Kernel, and the communication is done mainly using the MQTT protocol.

5.4 Novel Services Based on BLE Capabilities

5.4.1 Introduction to BLE Multiloop Communication Capabilities

The RADIO project identified the popularity that BLE attracts and foresees the benefits that modern IoT and Ambient Assisted Living (AAL) application domains will gain from the upcoming BLE mesh networking support. Therefore, RADIO designs a mesh mechanism that will be integrated in distributed sensor/actuator devices scattered across the RADIO AAL environment.

Network Formation

After a, thorough study of the existing approaches, the RADIO BLE mesh networking mechanism focused on the principles of BLE connectionless communications through advertising and scanning.

Advertising is the act of broadcasting data and it aims in device discovery and data publishing. The advertising mechanism involves two possible types of data packets that can be transmitted. The mandatory packet is the advertising packet while a node can optionally send a Scan Response packet. These two types of packets are structured mainly by the advertiser address and 31 bytes of payload as presented in Fig. 5.10. During the normal operation, the BLE advertiser constantly broadcasts the advertising packets within an advertising interval bounded by a minimum and maximum value. These intervals typically may range from 20 ms to 10.24 s.

During the network formation phase, the RADIO mesh mechanism utilizes the advertisement packets along with the broadcasting technique in order to achieve the network formation and route discovery. During the initialization of the network, each node broadcasts an advertising packet, which is the route discovery packet (route request—RREQ) in the context of the RADIO mesh. The RREQ messages are forwarded by each adjacent node until a pair of nodes exchange RREQs. Then a RREP message which contains the repliers address is sent backwards. During the reception of the RREPs, the respective neighbors table of each node is built. An instance of the neighbors table construction is presented in Fig. 5.11.

This flooding approach replicates every message at every relay node and is expected to deliver near optimal delivery probability. Furthermore, it does not require any knowledge about the network during the design time. The increased resource consumption can be tolerated since flooding occurs once during the network initialization. Furthermore, the deployment scale of the RADIO mesh network is not expected to expand more than a number of nodes for a small to medium

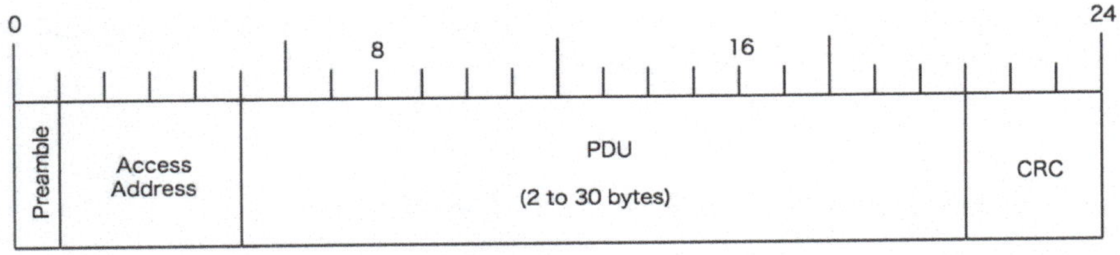

Fig. 5.10 Advertisement/scan response packets' structure

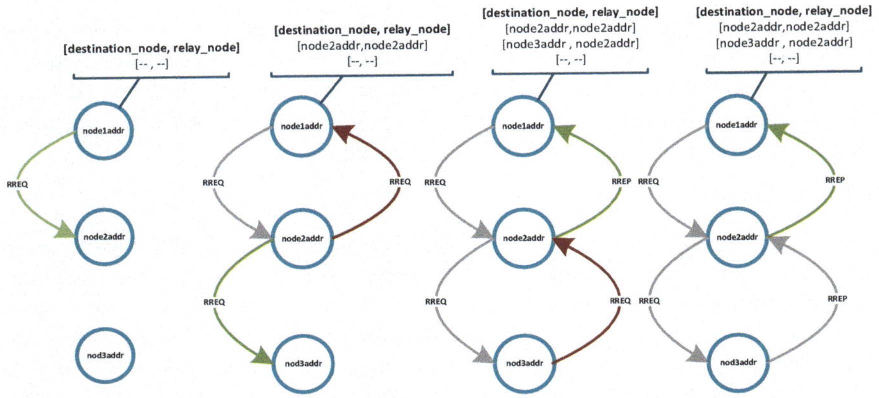

Fig. 5.11 Network discovery mechanism

network size. Scalability is accomplished since the route discovery can be performed on a new node's entrance.

Message Forwarding

After the network discovery is completed by every node of the network every node has knowledge about its surrounding neighbors. The nodes now are ready to start forwarding their data messages. The approach followed in every version of BLE mesh released by the industry so far is on the connectionless mode of BLE and advertisements are used as data carriers.

The first approach of the RADIO mesh forwards data messages through rebroadcasting. Rebroadcasting works by flooding all messages to all nodes in the network through broadcasts. Nodes are in scanning mode and when an advertisement is received, the receiver rebroadcasts it to its neighbors (Fig. 5.11). The process is repeated on every node and it is completed when every node receives the respective message. To avoid the broadcast storms through the continuously rebroadcasting of the same message, a versioning mechanism is implemented and runs on every receiver node. Upon the generation of the message on the source node, a version indicator is paired with the respective value and propagated along the network. Each relay node that receives the message stores it in a local data table.

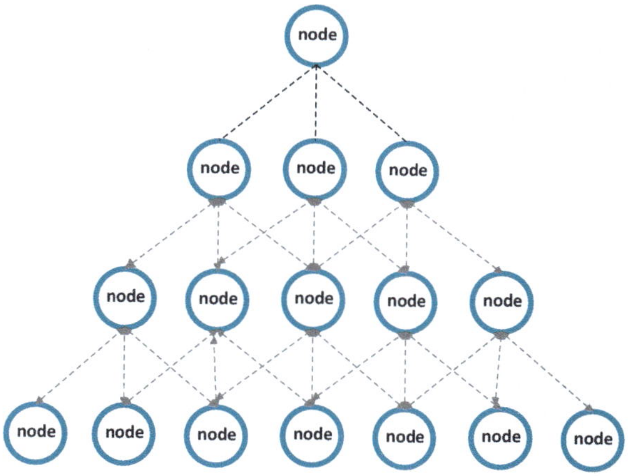

Fig. 5.12 Message forwarding with broadcasting

On every reception of a message from the same source and sensor, the relay node checks the version of the packet and propagates it to its neighbors if the received message version differs from the local. The message broadcasting process is completed when every node in the network received the message.

While broadcasting may increase the packet delivery ratio due to route redundancy it has a major drawback which highly affects the network performance under various network traffic loads and node density. Bluetooth Smart uses 40 RF channels in the ISM band (2.4 GHz). These RF channels have center frequencies $2402 + k * 2$ MHz where k ranges from 0 to 39. Advertising utilizes three of them specifically channel 37 (2402 MHz), 38 (2426 MHz) and 39 (2480 MHz). Due to broadcasting, the network is flooded with redundant transmissions. Thus, the poor utilization of frequency bands may degrade network performance and overall power consumption.

During the development and evaluation phase of the RADIO mesh a selective broadcasting policy was implemented. As described earlier, during the network phase, the nodes discover their neighbors and they store this knowledge locally. This knowledge is used to build the respective forwarding mechanism depending on the destination of their transmissions. These routing tables are used by the RADIO mesh to perform the selective broadcasting mechanism. The 29 bytes of payload are used to encapsulate the address of the destination node, the sensor model (described by the data type and data value) and the message version (described later). The application domain where RADIO mesh is deployed handles simple numeric sensor values that do not demand large packet payloads to carry them through the network. Therefore, the 29 bytes of the BLE advertisement packet is considered adequate for similar applications.

During the operation of the RADIO mesh with the selective broadcast enabled, every parent node that receives a message by the child node parses the payload of the packet and checks the packet's destination node. If the destination node is registered in its routing table, the message is rebroadcasted to its neighbors. In case

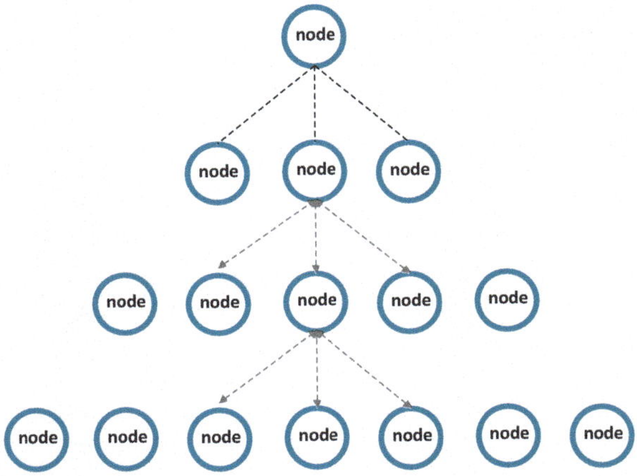

Fig. 5.13 Message forwarding with selective broadcasting

the relay node does not retrieve a route to the destination node it discards the packet from its queue. Figure 5.12 and give a visual representation of the traffic generated by the broadcasting and selective broadcasting transmissions. The figures show how the traffic load differentiates among the two approaches. Particularly we observe that selective broadcast relaxes the traffic load significantly, while at the same time retains a degree of route redundancy that benefits the packet delivery ratio without abusing the network resources (Fig. 5.13).

5.4.2 *Indoor Localization Based on BLE Beacons*

The following subsections outline a set of functionalities that must be efficiently executed on the robot platform focusing on the navigation functionality [18].

One fundamental problem in robotics is the simultaneous localization and mapping (SLAM), also known as Concurrent Mapping and Localization (CML) [13]. It arises when neither a map of the surrounding, nor the actual position of the robot is known. Several algorithms such as the SLAM with Extended Kalman Filters (EKF) and the SLAM with Particle Filters address this issue. The robot simultaneously creates a map of the environment and localizes itself relatively to this map. Within the RADIO project, a SLAM algorithm is implemented enabling self-localization estimation of the robot within the smart home. Based on the results of the SLAM algorithm, the robot is aware of its own position and can further use this information to navigate autonomously through the environment. This objective creates new challenges for man–machine interaction, as the robot should never become an obstacle for the human. Additionally, the robot is required to autonomously start the mapping process in "out-of-the-box" mode, meaning that it should detect by itself that its surroundings are unknown. When this detection is completed, the robot should start the mapping process. When autonomously mapping

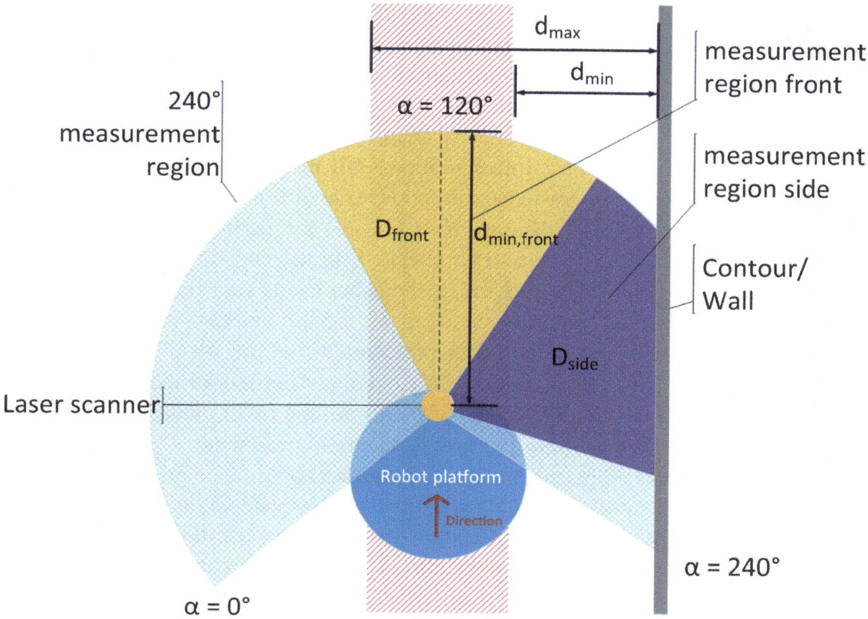

Fig. 5.14 Schematic process of following the contours

the surroundings, the robot will follow a contour (e.g., a wall) and chart the unknown environment with the data of the laser scanner and of its odometric sensors. Figure 5.15 shows the results of the mapping process. Figure 5.14 shows the robots mapping process.

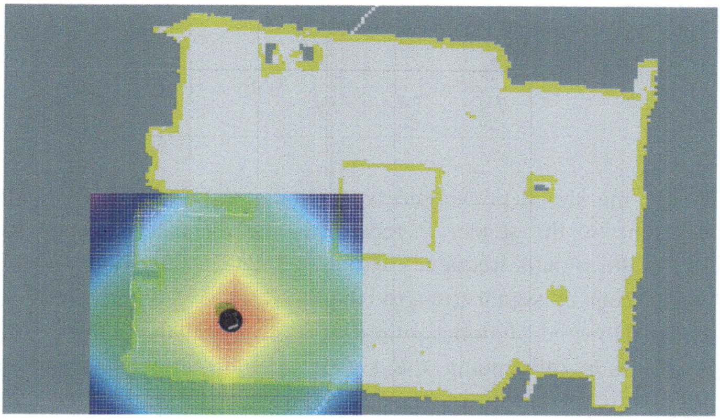

Fig. 5.15 Mapped exemplary room and estimated position of the robot

The robot platform will periodically measure the distances d_i between itself and the contour. The angle α represents the measurement angle corresponding to the measured distance. Based on α, the distances d_i are assigned to the region D_{front}, D_{side}, or are ignored. Figure 5.14 depicts D_{front} as a yellow and D_{side} as a purple region. If all $d_i \in D_{\text{side}}$ lie in the interval $[d_{\min}, d_{\max}]$ and all $d_i \in D_{\text{front}}$ are larger than $d_{\max}$, the robot performs a linear motion until the next measurement is initiated. The interval serves as hysteresis function to avoid the oscillation around the boundary limits $d_{\max}$ and $d_{\min}$. If some $d_i \in D_{\text{side}}$ do not lie in the interval, the two cases $d_i \leq d_{\min}$ and $d_i \geq d_{\max}$ have to be checked. In the case of $d_i \leq d_{\min}$ he robot has to turn left and in the case of $d_i \geq d_{\max}$ the robot has to turn right. This action is performed by changing the angular velocity ω. Additionally, if at least one $d_i \in D_{\text{front}}$ is smaller than $d_{\text{min,front}}$, the robot performs a rotation of $\omega > 0$ in order to avoid a frontal collision. This case generally occurs in corners of the room. After a finite amount of time, based on the size of the room, the robot created a map and is now able to localize itself within the now known environment.

Localization is very important for the cognition task since it provides the most relevant data regarding current distances to obstacles for safe navigation through the environment. The localization task depends on the data from the perception task. For localization within the SLAM algorithm, a particle filter can be chosen since it easily incorporates information from different sensor types, thus enabling sensor data fusion.

With additional sensors, the robot is also able to localize other objects. This can be accomplished with the Bluetooth devices that are positioned within the house. Thus, the robot can also help the end-user to search for an item which is outfitted with a BLE transmitter. Because Bluetooth beacons only broadcast their ID, the received signal strength indication (RSSI) is used in order to extract position information out of the beacons signal. The RSSI value can then be converted into a distance measurement. With one beacon, a distance measurement can only define a region of interest in which the receiver is currently located. The BLE receiver can extract a distance to the BLE beacons by solving the free space loss equation. In general the free space loss of a signal is described by

$$F = \frac{P_{\text{Rx}}}{P_{\text{Tx}}} = \left(\frac{\lambda}{4 \cdot \pi \cdot r}\right)^2, \text{with } \lambda = \frac{c}{f} \tag{5.1}$$

P_{Rx} indicates the signal power received by the receiver and P_{Tx} indicates the signal power sent by the sender. r represents the distance between sender and receiver and f is the signals frequency which is 2.4 GHz for Bluetooth. According to Eq. (5.1), the received signal strength is reduced by $\sim \frac{1}{r^2}$ with increasing distance from the sender. However, indoor environments vary greatly in terms of floor plan and equipment, thus influencing the signal strength through signal reflection, refraction, or interference with other signals. In order to incorporate these factors into the distance measurement, a logarithmic distance loss model is used. This

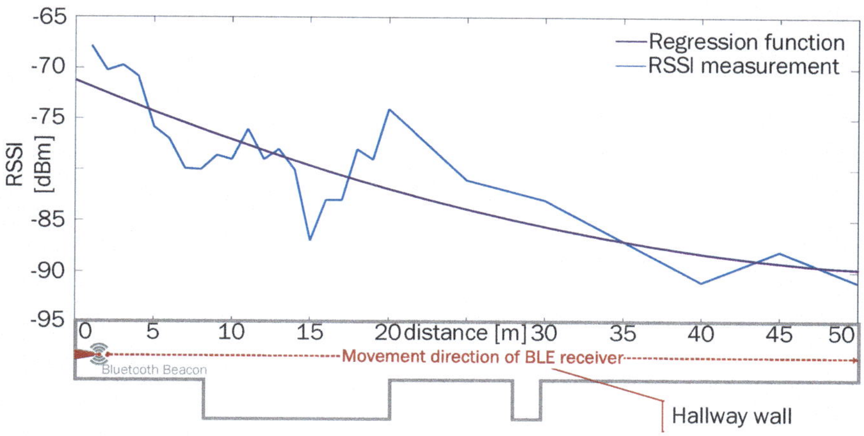

Fig. 5.16 RSSI to distance relation of in the hallway

model adds the variable γ which describes the signal loss in dependence on the surroundings [14].

$$\frac{P_{\mathrm{Rx}}}{\mathrm{dBm}} = \frac{P_0}{\mathrm{dBm}} - 10 \cdot \gamma \cdot \log_{10}\left(\frac{r}{r_0}\right), \text{with } \gamma \in R \tag{5.2}$$

Here, P_0 corresponds to the received signal strength to the corresponding distance r_0. The value for γ is determined through several test measurements with known distances. However, when using Eq. (5.2) for distance calculation, the resulting distances are very noisy and inaccurate. Therefore, converting the RSSI values into distances requires exhaustive measurements in the respective indoor environment because the absorption of the signal varies greatly depending on the surroundings.

Thus, the relation between RSSI values and the corresponding distance for our specific environment is effectively approximated. Because the relation of RSSI to distance is dependent on the surroundings, we performed measurements in a hallway which is 2 m wide and 50 m long and in a room with 4 m × 5 m floor space. Figure 5.16 shows the relation of RSSI and distance and the corresponding floorplan of the hallway.

A beacon was positioned at the start of the hallway in 1.5 m height; see Fig. 5.16 the red icon on the left. Starting from the beacons position, signal strength measurements are conducted in 1-m intervals until the end of the hallway is reached. At every measurement position, 40 individual measurements are acquired, and the mean value is calculated. All measured mean RSSI values are shown by the blue line in Fig. 5.16. Between 8 m and 20 m, a larger width of the hallway can be seen. In this region, the RSSI values do not correlate well to their respective distance. We can see a decrease of the received signal power from −79 to

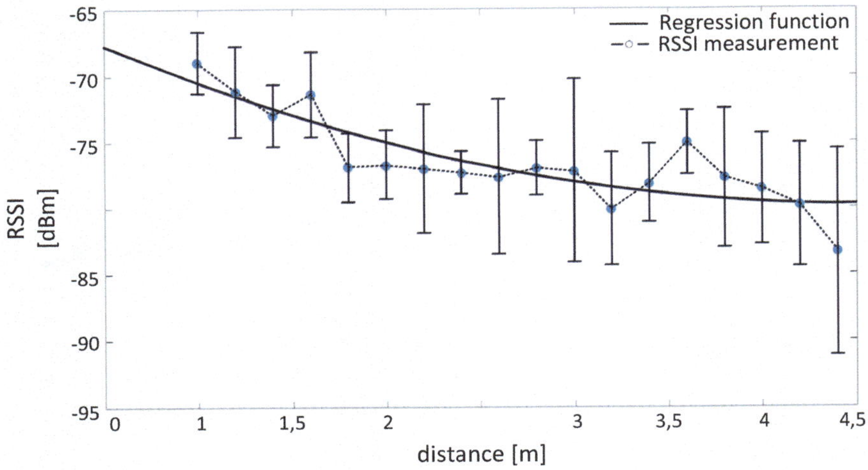

Fig. 5.17 RSSI to distance relation of the 4 m × 5 m room

−87 dBm. This occurrence leads to the assumption that in this region more reflections and refractions influence the signal strength. In the region after 20 m distance, the signal power increases again to −73 dBm. As can be seen, no direct relation between the RSSI values and the corresponding distance can be established. The RSSI values do not even decrease monotonously with increasing distance. Therefore, we determine a regression function which fits the measurements in a satisfactory manner. The regression function is depicted in Eq. (5.3)

$$r(x_{\text{rssi}}) = 0.07472 \cdot x_{\text{rssi}}^2 + 10.106 \cdot x_{\text{rssi}} + 345.21 \tag{5.3}$$

The measurements in the 4 m × 5 m room show a different behavior of the signal strength in relation to the respective distance. Figure 5.17 shows the RSSI to distance relation of the 4 m × 5 m room.

For each position, 200 measurements were performed. The deviation of an individual measurement can be up to 11% from the mean value over all 200 measurements. The standard deviation of the respective measurement point is depicted in Fig. 5.17 as bar plot. The regression function which fits the measurements best is shown in Eq. (5.4).

$$r(x_{\text{rssi}}) = 0.0010332 \cdot x_{\text{rssi}}^3 0.24022 \cdot x_{\text{rssi}}^2 + 18.32 \cdot x_{\text{rssi}} + 460.89 \tag{5.4}$$

With no further information, the distance r describes a sphere in 3D space, see Eq. (5.5).

$$(x - x_m)^2 + (y - y_m)^2 + (z - z_m)^2 = r^2, \tag{5.5}$$

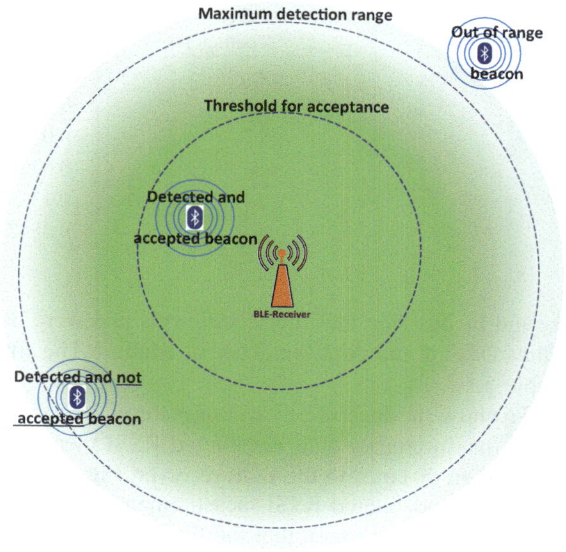

Fig. 5.18 Thresholding of range determined through the RSSI values of BLE beacons

with $(x_m, y_m z_m)$ being the BLE receivers position. This 3D problem can be reduced to a 2D problem, by assuming that the height z_B of the beacons is known. Thus, the sphere can be reduced to a circle. The circle has the center at $(x_m, y_m z_B)$ and the resulting radius can be calculated as

$$r_C = \sqrt{r^2 - (z_m - z_B)^2}. \tag{5.6}$$

Thus we can describe every possible position of a BLE beacon through

$$\begin{bmatrix} x \\ y \end{bmatrix} = \begin{bmatrix} x_m + r_C \cos \varphi \\ y_m + r_C \cos \varphi \end{bmatrix} \text{ with } 0 \leq \varphi \leq 2\pi \tag{5.7}$$

Through thresholding of the beacons measured distance, simple annotation of regions within an indoor environment is possible. This approach is shown in Fig. 5.18.

The main problem with this approach is that the RSSI values are very noisy. Because of the RSSI noisy properties, a single RSSI measurement does not yield accurate and therefore valuable information. Therefore, some manner of prefiltering has to be executed before the distance conversion. As a prefilter, we use a 10th order finite impulse response (FIR) filter. The FIR filter equation is shown in Eq. (5.8).

$$y_n = \frac{1}{a_0} \left\{ \sum_{k=0}^{N} b_k \cdot x_{n-k} \right\} \tag{5.8}$$

Table 5.1 Fir filter coefficients

Filter coefficients	Value	Filter coefficients	Value
a_0	1	b_5	0.3071
b_0	−0.0349	b_6	0.2562
b_1	−0.0370	b_7	0.1368
b_2	0.0209	b_8	0.02092
b_3	0.1368	b_9	−0.0370
b_4	0.2562	b_{10}	−0.0349

a_0 and b_k describe the filter coefficients and were determined with the help of the Filter Design and Analysis Tool of Matlab. The filter coefficients are depicted in Table 5.1.

To show the increase in accuracy through the above filter, we compare the raw RSSI measurements with the filtered RSSI measurements. A beacon is positioned with 1.2 m distance to the BLE receiver. Figure 5.19 shows the different results of raw RSSI and filtered RSSI measurements.

It can be clearly seen that the filtered RSSI measurements are more stable than the raw RSSI measurements. To further evaluate the performance of the filtered RSSI measurement approach, we perform RSSI measurements in a radius of 1.2 m distance of the BLE beacon, see Fig. 5.20. 150 measurements were acquired on the circle in order to examine the behavior of the RSSI values when the transceiver has the same distance to the BLE beacon but a different orientation.

When calculating the distance out of the filtered RSSI values with Eq. (5.4), the mean value for the calculated distance is approximately 1.1 m with a standard deviation of 0.054 m. This results in a nominal error to the true distance of 10 cm or 8.3%. Since the uncertainty of the calculated distances is in the range of single

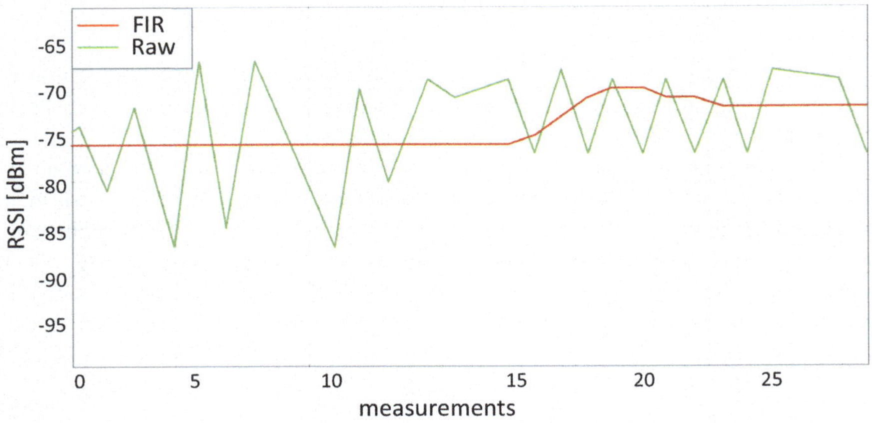

Fig. 5.19 Comparison of raw RSSI data and FIR filtered RSSI data

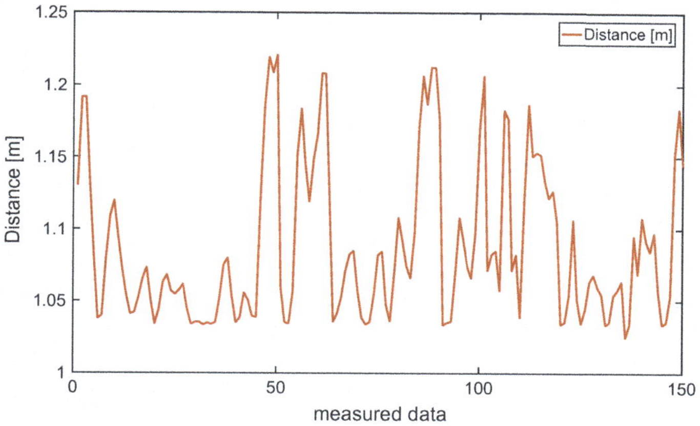

Fig. 5.20 Calculated distance out of filtered RSSI measurements. 150 Measurements were performed in a circle with 1.2 m radius distance to the BLE beacon

digit centimeters, accurate position estimation with several RSSI measurements can be performed.

For accurate position estimation through trilateration, three measurements at different positions have to be performed. Each position generates a circle with a certain radius which describes the measured distance to the BLE beacon. In the case of three measurement positions, 27 circle constellations exist. These 27 constellations contain redundant constellations which do not need to be analyzed separately. Then, these 27 constellations can be reduced to 10 different circle arrangements. We assume that no circle is contained within another circle except if several measurement errors occur. Therefore, we discard the circle arrangements where circles are included in other circles. Then, we receive four valid arrangements as seen in Fig. 5.21. They are used to determine the region of interest (ROI) with the help of multi-lateration [15].

In the first arrangement, each circle has no intersection with the other circles. In this case, the center of the shortest connection for every circle pair is determined. These three calculated points are the triangle out of which the position estimation can be calculated for the BLE beacon. The region of interest is the circumcircle of the triangle with the radius being the uncertainty of the measurement.

In the second arrangement, exactly two circles intersect with each other. Then two intersection points exist. One of the intersection points has a larger distance to the third circle than the other intersection point. The intersection point with the larger distance is discarded and the resulting region of interest is a circle with the center point being the center of the shortest connection between the remaining intersection point and the third circle while the radius of the circle and thus the uncertainty is half the length of the connection.

In the third arrangement, one circle serves as connector to the two other circles. The two other circles do not share any intersection while the circle in the middle has

Fig. 5.21 Four possible circle arrangements

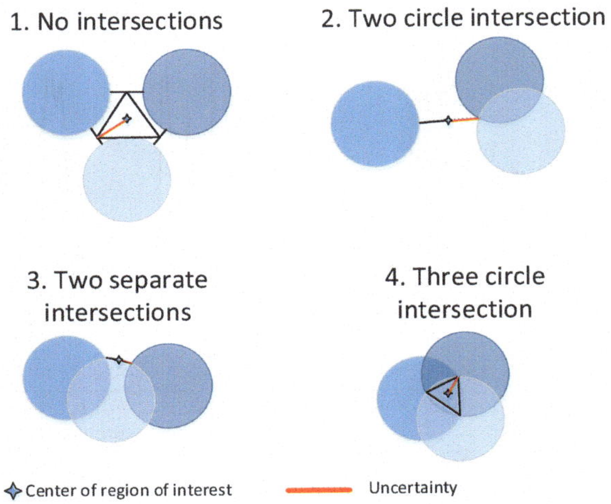

two intersections with the respective circle. In order to determine the region of interest, all intersection points have to be calculated and the four distances between the intersection point pairs from the different circles have to be determined. The intersection point pair with the smallest distance is chosen and the center of this connection is the center point of the region of interest circle with the radius being half the length of the connection.

In the fourth arrangement, all circles intersect with each other. The distance to the remaining circle is calculated for each intersection point. The intersection point with smallest distance to the remaining circle is chosen as final point for the resulting triangle. Just as in the first case, our region of interest is formed by the circumcircle of the resulting triangle.

If more than three measurements are performed, this approach is also valid. Then we consider four triples of circles (1, 2, 3), (1, 2, 4), (1, 3, 4), and (2, 3, 4) separately. The triple with the smallest measurement error determines then the final region of interest.

5.5 Backend Infrastructures

5.5.1 EnConrtol

The smart home architecture in RADIO is based on a white label B2B product by Sensing & Control Systems called *enControl*™. *enControl*™ provided an initial solution for home automation, and was enhanced and upgraded complementing other technologies and developments within RADIO in order to build the final RADIO solution. The main four functionalities[1] of *enControl*™ are

(1) Comfort
   a. Climate monitoring
   b. Climate control
   c. Temperature, Humidity, CO_2 (etc.) levels
(2) Security
   a. Detection of door/window opening
   b. Detection of movement
   c. Detection of Smoke
   d. Detection of CO
   e. Detection of water basement
(3) Energy Management
   a. Energy consumption
   b. Energy control (switch on/off electricity, water, gas, etc.)
(4) Automation
   a. Switch on/off appliances
   b. Switch on/off lights
   c. Open/Close doors, curtains, shutters.

Smart home backend is divided into two main components, (i) home devices, and (ii) IoT Platform. The home devices component includes sensors, actuators and the home controller. The home controller is a product from Sensing & Control that complements the smart home functions delivered by the IoT platform. The IoT platform contains the core of the smart home solution. It provides an open REST API enabling the home controllers to exchange information bi-directionally, based on synchronous or asynchronous actions triggered by IoT and/or end-users through *enControl*™ interfaces. Also, the IoT platform acts as an information repository, storing both historical data about sensors (values and status) and actions triggered by users, enabling to know what action was executed, by who, and when. For example, "the TV set has been switched on by Maria on 11 July 2015, 20:30 CET".

The IoT platform is able to connect, transport, process, analyze, and manage data from the sensors to the real world to high-level applications and vice versa. It is able to operate in both wireless/wired network environments and supports different communication protocols. As a function summary

[1]The list does not pretend to cover all possibilities, the Reader should understand that the smart home solution can integrate any Z-WAVE standard product, thus enabling the functionality delivered by a particular product. For full list of product, please visit Z-WAVE alliance web page.

- **Collect data**
  Collect data refers to the ability to retrieve and store information for further exploitation about all the parameters that are relevant to the system: messages, device status, commands, errors, exceptions.
- **Analyze data**
  The IoT Platform has processes in charge of analyzing data and taking decisions based on the quality/importance/integrity of this data.
- **Data Aggregation/Data Fusion**
  Data aggregation refers to the ability to concatenate info from devices, for example when there is a mix of information between data from mash-up sensors. Data fusion, is the process of integration of multiple data and knowledge representing the same real-world object into a consistent, accurate, and useful representation.
- **Translate data**
  This feature is related to the ability to transform raw data in bytes from the devices to high-level information.
- **System monitor**
  The IoT Platform is able to monitor the communication between devices and high-level apps; and the overall status of the platform and device network. For instance, it is used to monitor key performance indicators like the number of messages sent per minute, number of exceptions/errors, number of devices connected to the platform, etc.
- **Transfer**
  The platform provides mechanisms to publish subscribe information to the queues exposed by the SDK.
- **Audit information**
  In order to enable traceability of the functionality of all subsystems, active logging is implemented within the software components. Log files are stored and available for analysis.
- **Secure components and communications**
  Communication between components and devices are secured.

The current solution of *enControl*™ provides means of interaction with home devices by accessing dedicated functions of the open API of the IoT platform. This implies that other ICT solutions (either at home like other RADIO components or remotely) willing to interact with *enControl*™ must have Internet connection (Fig. 5.22).

The API is divided into following main groups:

(1) Authorisation and Authentication
    Functions used to grant access to different IoT resources and API functions
(2) Devices
    Functions related to push and retrieve device status and data (including historical data)

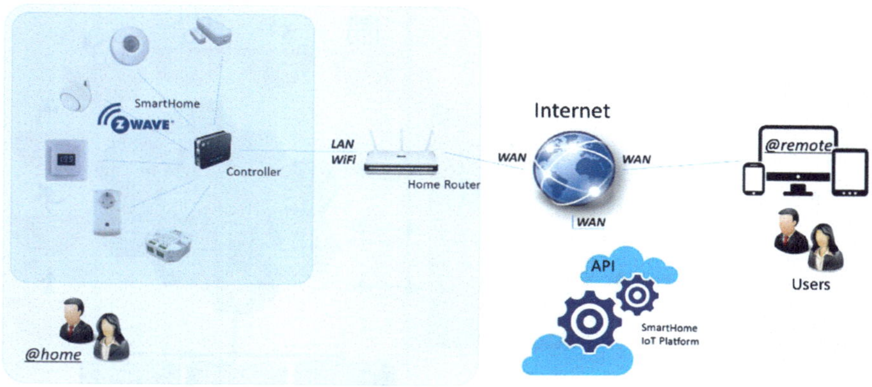

Fig. 5.22 enControl™ service architecture

(3) Users
 Functions related to the management of users
(4) Installations
 Functions related to the management of smart home installations
(5) Monitor
 Functions related to the status monitoring of the IoT

The open REST API is used by user interfaces through web clients and smartphone apps in order to present to end-users the information being acquired from home end devices, and the action than can be triggered to them, so it encapsulates the smart home functions offered.

It is important to notice that *enControl*™ clients (smartphone apps and Web interfaces, third-party services, etc.) interact with the smart home through the API, making Internet connections required. It should be noted that experience with deployment of the solution is that this introduces no perceptible delay in executing actions by Z-Wave devices.

5.5.2 ATLAS Presentation

In this section, a conceptual analysis of the ATLAS IoT platform as the technician's backend platform in the context of RADIO project is presented. Starting from the left-hand side of Fig. 5.23, an efficient, flexible, and extendible approach is targeted so that any kind of heterogeneous sensor or actuation modality is aggregated at the ATLAS Gateway. In order to support the heterogeneity posed by different wireless communication technologies, the MQTT-SN [16] protocol, has been selected, as a prominent communication protocol.

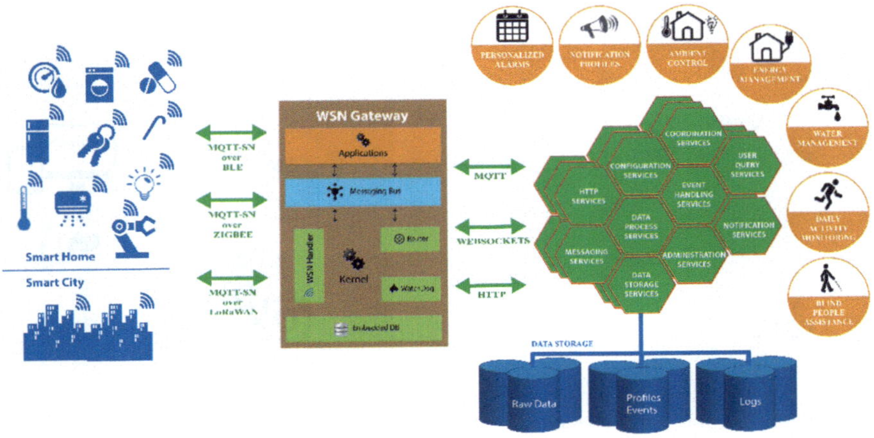

Fig. 5.23 ATLAS IoT platform

MQTT-SN is a publish/subscribe messaging protocol that extends the well-established Message Queue Telemetry Transport (MQTT) [17] protocol in order to cope with the specific constraints of WSNs, such as resource-limited and battery-operated devices, low network bandwidth and high link failures. Another critical conceptual choice, designing such IoT platforms, concerns the way data, events or/and commands can be exchanged between the Gateway and the backend infrastructure. In that respect, ATLAS IoT Platform, besides the well-known HTTP protocol, expose additional communication interfaces, such as MQTT and WebSockets, in order to consume real time data from multiple sources, from both indoor and outdoor environments.

In the core of ATLAS platform, the deployed services are based on the microservices architectural pattern, which allows to deploy small autonomous applications, that states on the single responsibility principle. Using this architectural pattern, ATLAS services can be deployed and scaled independently in the ATLAS Cloud Infrastructure, without affecting the overall performance of the platform.

Finally, given the growing needs for data-driven features and the complexity of modern IoT applications, it is important to offer services able to share and store data in an isolated and scalable way. In that respect, at the bottom level of the architecture, ATLAS IoT Platform deploys a heterogeneous data storage system, consisting from multiple different storage types, such as SQL, NoSQL, Key-Value stores, etc., to address the diversity of data. On top of the deployed databases, ATLAS IoT Platform implements an abstraction layer that provides simplified data access using simple APIs to hide completely the complexity posed by database heterogeneity and low-level mechanisms for data manipulation.

5.6 Summary

This chapter aims to highlight multifaceted experience and knowledge gained in the context of RADIO project, from the efforts devoted to offer a reliable, efficient, and versatile end-to-end communication infrastructure. Therefore, initially the conceptual architecture is clearly presented which, in conjunction with the application scenarios, effectively drove the identification of adequate requirements that the end solution should meet. As indicated, such requirements span over a wide range of challenging and diverse demands concerning both the Wireless Sensor Network domain but also the backend communication infrastructure.

Then, the main ultra-low power wireless communication technologies selected, supported and integrated by the RADIO communication platform are presented highlighting critical characteristics and features for the RADIO communication objectives. One of the main characteristics of the RADIO communication platform is efficient and seamless support of heterogenous communication protocols. Towards this goal in the context of the RADIO concept the Gateway device is of cornerstone importance since it comprises the entity that effectively supports all different communication paradigm and offers a unified way of data transfer from and to the sensors. Therefore, critical aspects of this compound component are presented in detail in Sect. 5.3.

However, in RADIO significant effort is devoted on offer extended and enhanced features and functionalities related to the adopted communication technologies. Therefore, in Sect. 5.4, two such endeavors are indicated. On one hand, attempt to extend the BLE protocol to support multi-hop communication is presented while, on the other hand, indoor localization techniques based on BLE sensors are analyzed.

Last but not least, the backend communication infrastructure technologies adopted and exploited in RADIO project, also comprising critical cornerstones to meet the overall project's objectives are presented in Sect. 5.5.

References

1. Giannakopoulos, T., Konstantopoulos, S., Siantikos, G., & Karkaletsis, V. (2016). Design for a system of multimodal interconnected ADL recognition services. In *Components and services for IoT platforms: Paving the way for IoT standards.* Berlin: Springer (Reproduced as Chap. 2 of this volume).
2. On developing a novel versatile framework for heterogeneous home monitoring WSN networks. http://www.ingentaconnect.com/content/doaj/24117145/2015/00000001/00000001/ art00005.
3. http://ec.europa.eu/information_society/newsroom/cf/dae/document.cfm?action=display& doc_ id= 7681.
4. http://www.cloud-council.org/deliverables/CSCC-Cloud-Customer-Architecture-for-IoT.pdf.
5. http://www.shimmersensing.com/.
6. https://www.movisens.com/en/.
7. *Revoking Networks "advanced user manual"*, version 4.77 2/3/2011.

8. https://wiki.csr.com/wiki/CSRmesh.
9. https://github.com/NordicSemiconductor/nRF51-ble-bcast-mesh.
10. Philip, L., et al. (2011). The trickle algorithm. No. RFC 6206.
11. https://github.com/openthread/openthread.
12. Bluetooth, SIG (Hrsg.): Specification of the bluetooth system: Covered core package version: 4.0, June 2010.
13. Thrun, S., Burgard, W., & Fox, D. *Probabilistic robotics*. MA: The MIT Press. ISBN: 978-0-262-20162-9.
14. Grossmann, U., Schauch, M., & Hakobyan, S. (2007). The accuracy of algorithms for WLAN indoor positioning and the standardization of signal reception for different mobile devices. *International Journal of Computing, 6*(1), 103–109.
15. Kuruoglu, G. S., Erol, M., & Oktug S. (2009). Localization in wireless sensor networks with range measurement errors. In *Fifth Advanced International Conference on Telecommunications*, Istanbul.
16. Andy Stan-ford-Clark and Hong Linh Truong—MQTT for sensor networks (MQTT-SN) protocol specification, version 1.2. http://mqtt.org/new/wp-content/uploads/2009/06/MQTT-SN_spec_v1.2.pdf (November 2013).
17. MQTT Protocol Specification. http://docs.oasis-open.org/mqtt/mqtt/v3.1.1/os/mqtt-v3.1.1-os.pdf (29 October, 2014).
18. Schwiegelshohn, F., Wehner, P., Werner, F., Göhringer, D., & Hübner, M. (2016). Enabling in-door object localization through bluetooth beacons on the RADIO robot platform. In *Proceedings of the International Conference on Embedded Computer Systems: Architectures, Modeling and Simulation (SAMOS XV)*, Samos, Greece, (pp. 1–6).

Chapter 6
ROS as Integration Medium for Service Robotics

Georgios Stavrinos and Román Navarro García

6.1 The Robot Operating System

6.1.1 Advantages

Open Source: Robot Operating System (ROS) is an open-source project, which means that its source code is available for use and modification. Open-source software leads to quicker development due to its open nature, in which anyone can contribute. It is also much easier for a big group of developers to debug problematic code in comparison to a fairly small development group of a company.

Big community: ROS has become the most used robotic framework of all time. Its downloads reached almost 14 million and its unique users are almost 250 thousand just in 2017.[1]

With such big community, a lot of robotics applications have already been implemented, enhancing the availability of ready-to-use software. Even if an already implemented method does not fit exactly the requirements of a project, it offers a codebase that can be used for further development, expansion of its capabilities and integration.

Hardware Drivers: ROS offers a wide variety of hardware drivers from simple motors and webcams, to robotic arms, stereoscopic cameras, laser scanners, and

[1]https://discourse.ros.org/t/the-2017-ros-metrics-report/2659/2.

G. Stavrinos (✉)
Institute of Informatics and Telecommunications, NCSR "Demokritos", Aghia Paraskevi, Greece
e-mail: gstavrinos@iit.demokritos.gr

R. N. García
Robotnik Automation, SLL, Valencia, Spain
e-mail: rnavarro@robotnik.es

V. Karkaletsis et al. (eds.), *RADIO–Robots in Assisted Living*,
https://doi.org/10.1007/978-3-319-92330-7_6

more. The wide variety of hardware driver availability enables ROS users to customize their robots based on their needs and budget.

Hardware Agnostic: In addition to the wide variety of hardware drivers, the architecture of ROS provides hardware abstraction, meaning that developed methods can work on different robots without modification. This boosts the reusability of code, and saves development time for already implemented methods.

Basic functions are available out of the box: ROS installation comes with a series of default software capabilities (packages). Those packages include robot simulation and visualization tools, as well as implementations of popular methods like ALCL localization and shortest path planning with the Dijkstra and A* algorithms. The available functionality which can always be expanded and improved by the ROS community makes it easier to launch a project.

Modular: Software written using ROS is modular. Each part of the software is considered a stand-alone component that should have the ability to be used with other ROS components. The modularity of the software written using ROS offers extreme flexibility on software usage and allows for easy plugging and unplugging of software components without affecting the rest of the system.

Distributed: The main advantage of the ROS core functionality is its ability to handle software as a distributed system of processes. Running software on one or multiple machines does not require different methodologies either to use or develop software.

6.1.2 Disadvantages

Steep learning curve: ROS comes in a variety of versions for different operating systems and offers a significant amount of available software to use. It is based on a series of standards and expects software to be developed and packaged in certain ways. All these can be really overwhelming for new users, and even experienced users sometimes struggle through the complexity of its awesomeness.

Sometimes unstable: ROS is being actively developed by programmers all over the world, but it is not supported financially by a company so it does not follow company standards, at least not as strictly. Software development companies make sure that their delivered software is always in stable condition, bug free and unit tested. Although the core components of ROS are almost always stable and bug free, the same cannot be said for external ROS packages that have been implemented by the community. Most of the times, overcoming problems encountered in ROS software is easy, given that the software was intended for the ROS version that is being used. This leads us to the final problem with ROS.

A lot of ROS releases: Every year a new ROS version is released, mainly with small, but sometimes with also big, changes to the core components. Every two years a new LTS version is released. This cycle of releases follows the releases of Ubuntu Linux. This release matching also means that each new release of ROS supports mainly the new Ubuntu Linux version. Switching to a newer version of the used operating system to support the latest ROS version is a requirement that for some projects, apart from time consuming, is also impossible, since the access to the hardware might be limited, or the implemented software has other requirements that would be unmet with an upgrade. This vicious circle continues, since packages developed using a certain ROS version need to undergo zero to highly impactful changes to support other ROS releases.

6.1.3 Typical Usage

The most typical usage of a ROS installation requires only a robot that is equipped with a series of sensors and an onboard computer. All software is running on the onboard computer, hardware (sensor) drivers are publishing messages that are being transmitted to nodes and the latter are publishing results based on sensor inputs.

A more advanced but still typical use of a ROS installation is between two machines. One machine is the robot and the other one is a machine used for monitoring, being a desktop or a laptop. With those two machines connected on the same LAN, and a little configuration on both ends, they can run any number of nodes on either of the two machines without modification on the code. One of the two machines is running the ROS master node, which is responsible for, along with many other tasks, to manage message transmission to the correct nodes. Message information is always transmitted to the ROS master, and then a direct connection is established between the nodes that need to communicate.

Finally, a nonstandard method is the use of specific ROS packages that allow a multi-master configuration, where all the machines on the network are independent masters but they are connected and synchronized between them by means of these packages. This configuration is useful when the network communication is not reliable.

6.2 The RADIO ROS System

The RADIO system consists of a Turtlebot 2 equipped with an Intel NUC and an FPGA, three Raspberry Pis and an optional Android mobile device for the end user. From those, the Intel NUC, the FPGA, one of the Raspberry Pis and the mobile device are running ROS. From now on, the Raspberry Pi that is running ROS is going to be called the Main Controller. The other two Raspberry Pis are used for smart home events and object/robot localization using Bluetooth Low Energy (BLE) beacons. From now on, the Raspberry Pi running smart-home-related software is going to be called Smart Home (SH) Gateway, and the other one that is running BLE beacons-related software is going to be called BLE Gateway. The mobile device is used to send commands to the robot, control the smart home or receive various notifications. An abstract architecture of the RADIO ecosystem is shown below.

6.2.1 Communication Via ROS Topics

Topics are the main way to transfer and exchange data in ROS. Topics are like channels, on which everyone subscribed can receive all messages published to it. The main purpose of topics is sensor data streaming. In many circumstances though, a single message needs to be sent, to trigger a certain behavior.

Early versions of the RADIO system used topics for all kinds of data transmission. Since topics are intended for data streaming, messages are not guaranteed to be delivered to all of the subscribed nodes. In a ROS ecosystem with many devices and big bandwidth usage, lost messages are a very common problem, which is of vital importance when a message is only being sent once. One of the ideas that were discussed when this problem started making the whole system misbehave, was to create a TCP-like protocol, where a message would be sent until a response message was received by the original publisher, but this implementation apart from ugly, becomes too complicated when there are multiple subscribers that need to have a verification for successfully transferred messages.

6.2.2 Networking

ROS Networking is based on the ROS master node. As described earlier, the master node is responsible for creating connections between nodes that need to exchange messages. This means that without a master node the system cannot work. As a matter of fact, all ROS nodes fall into a loop waiting for a ROS master to be detected before initialization. During our tests, we learned that in a system where machines are moving (robots) and everything is connected on a home network, bandwidth and WiFi cannot be trusted and the overall system should always assume that something might get disconnected. A huge disadvantage of the ROS master architecture is that when a ROS node loses connection with the master, it will most probably crash, and will not recover when the connection with the master is restored. Although using WiFi repeaters could help broaden the WiFi coverage, messages could still be lost due to bandwidth limitations.

6.2.3 Localization

The robot uses a 2D localization system to map and localize through every home. The robot has mounted a 2D laser for this purpose as well as for navigation.

The algorithms and packages used are the ROS standard ones: slam_gmapping for mapping and amcl for localizing.

To set the initial pose of the robot (necessary for amcl), we used an AR tag that was conveniently placed and mapped in front of the robot's charging position. Every time the robot starts up, it reads the marker and updates the global pose of the robot.

6.2.4 Navigation

At first, our Turtlebot 2 used the typical ROS indoors navigation configuration to navigate through houses. The typical navigation stack, uses a global planner based on the Dijkstra's shortest path algorithm, and a local planner with obstacle avoidance capabilities. Although the out-of-the-box autonomous navigation capabilities offered in ROS are very robust, sometimes we encountered problems with people walking in corridors or furniture being moved. The main problem was the fact that an obstacle that was seen in the past, like a moving person, could no longer be in the same position that was marked on the robot's map, but the robot would still refuse to generate a path through that presently non-existent obstacle. Accumulatively these added false positives (obstacles) would block all routes to a robot's goal and the robot even though physically possible, would not be able to autonomously navigate and start spinning as part of its recovery behaviors until it would ultimately stop.

6.2.5 Node Handling

In the early versions of the RADIO system, we were using system calls through Python to start and stop nodes, by running "roslaunch", "rosrun", and "rosnode kill" commands. This method, although effective, did not give any clue of the result of the executed commands, and also the added of starting a node could result in losing valuable sensor data. In addition to all the previous problems, the "rosnode kill" command would sometimes not stop the requested node, adding unnecessary CPU load and also result in failed future executions of "roslaunch" or "rosrun" commands for that same node.

6.2.6 Bridging Various Devices and Protocols

As stated in the introduction the RADIO ecosystem, apart from the machines running ROS, it includes a Raspberry Pi that controls smart home sensors via the ZWave protocol and another one that runs the MQTT protocol for Bluetooth beacons. The Main Controller, which is the central unit for the purposes of the system, needed a way to extract the information from those two machines. For the BLE Gateway, a simple ROS-MQTT bridge was written just for the purposes of this specific task. The Smart Home Gateway was part of a commercial smart home solution so we did not have direct access to the ZWave data of the sensors. The Smart Home Gateway provided a JSON API for data extraction though, resulting in a ROS-JSON bridge that would extract JSON sensor data and ultimately publish them to a ROS topic.

6.2.7 First RADIO Architecture Summary

The first RADIO Architecture, even if partially working, it was not stable and effective enough. Messages through ROS Topics were lost, nodes would get disconnected from the master node and never recover, nodes would not start or stop properly and navigation would fail in seemingly trivial autonomy tasks.

The diagram below shows an abstract version of the architecture of the system. The red line shows the part with the major data loss problems.

6.3 Final Implementation

While working on improving the RADIO system, we found many ways to increase its stability. This chapter is very important, since it presents the final implementation that offered the best performance for the RADIO system. All of the methodologies followed could be applicable to any large-scale ROS project, and this chapter can be seen as a "cheatsheet" for many future projects.

6.3.1 Communication Via ROS Services

ROS Topics are a very straight forward way to transmit data from a node to many others (one to many). Their "streaming nature" though, does not guarantee message delivery, and this creates a lot of problems when only a single message can be sent. In order to be able to guarantee message delivery, all of the single message ROS Topics where switched over to ROS Services.

ROS Services guarantee delivery but can only connect one node with another (one to one). This creates the extra need for additional service calls, which is not a problem. With ROS Services a node that needs to send or get data from another node, calls a predefined service name, and checks if it is available first. If it is, everything is guaranteed to be delivered. If the node that serves the requested service is not available, the caller can wait some time and then report an error.

First checking if a service is available and then proceeding to use it is a workflow that ROS Services require and ensures that the overall system works as expected.

6.3.2 Rostune

While working on the various machines that are used in RADIO, we thought that we should be able to measure the overhead on each machine, to increase the overall performance. ROS does not provide such tool, so we implemented one.

Rostune is a package that generates statistics for CPU, RAM and network usage. The statistics are provided through the form of ROS messages and can be visualized with any of the visualization tools provided in ROS. PlotJuggler is especially effective in visualizing such data. With the help of the statistics provided by rostune, we were able to experiment with different distributions of our nodes to conclude on the most effective.

6.3.3 ROS Multimaster

A system based on the ROS master node architecture, although very effective, is very easy to collapse. A malfunction on the machine running the master node or the network, can cause the whole system to break down.

The best way to fix the master node problem is to use the multimaster ROS package. Multimaster uses an architecture in which two or more machines can run a master node, and all other node can connect to either of those masters. Losing connection is no problem, given that at least one master is available. When all machines are running a master, even if the network goes down, each machine will keep its nodes running, and reconnect to the other masters when the network is available again. In the RADIO system, the robot and the main controller are running a master, and the rest of the nodes are connected to those two machines. We could have a master run on each different machine, but the network instability was mainly between the robot and the main controller.

6.3.4 Navigation

Having the problems with non-existent obstacles that were seen in the past, we needed a way for the robot to check previous locations and try to navigate through them even. The easiest way to achieve this task was to force a costmap update every time the robot could not find a path to its goal. This solved all the problems with non-existent obstacles. Basically, this behavior can be achieved by adding the costmap clearing recovery behavior plugin to the navigation stack.

6.3.5 System Startup

Node management in the first implementations of the RADIO system was done through system commands. Using this method, processes do not always start or stop successfully, generating a lot of zombie processes, while at the same time decreasing the performance and effectiveness of the system.

The final approach on this matter was to always run all available nodes, but have them in an idle state. This was achieved by adding a service to all nodes that needed to be started and stopped under specific circumstances. Those ROS services could also report the current state of the node (running/idle). This added functionality enabled the system to always know the states of all its nodes, making increasing the overall stability and robustness.

6.4 Conclusion

The final implementation of the RADIO system was robust, and the methodologies and approaches presented above aided in achieving the desired stability.

Also, ROS was proven to be a wise choice both as integration middleware and as a pool of base components upon which to build the RADIO Robot software stack.

Chapter 7
Accelerating AAL Home Services Using Embedded Hardware Components

Georgios Keramidas, Christos P. Antonopoulos, Nikolaos S. Voros, Fynn Schwiegelshohn, Philipp Wehner, Michael Huebner, Diana Göhringer and Evaggelinos Mariatos

7.1 Introduction

RADIO aims to provide a real-life solution to support elderly people in their domestic environment [1]. The core concept and approach of the project has been presented in more details in [2]. It is important to note that the RADIO project emphasizes on being unobtrusive and well accepted while remaining fit for its clinical purpose. Technically, these requirements pertain to user interfacing, specifically adapted to the elderly; ethically and clinically adequate data collection,

G. Keramidas (✉) · C. P. Antonopoulos · N. S. Voros
Embedded System Design and Application Lab, Computer and Informatics Engineering Department, Technological Educational Institution of Western Greece, Patra, Greece
e-mail: gkeramidas@teiwest.gr

C. P. Antonopoulos
e-mail: cantonopoulos@teiwest.gr

N. S. Voros
e-mail: voros@teiwest.gr

F. Schwiegelshohn · P. Wehner · M. Huebner
Ruhr-University, Bochum, Germany
e-mail: fynn.schwiegelshohn@rub.de

P. Wehner
e-mail: philipp.wehner@rub.de

M. Huebner
e-mail: michael.huebner@rub.de

D. Göhringer
Technische Universitaet Dresden, Dresden, Germany
e-mail: diana.goehringer@tu-dresden.de

E. Mariatos
AVN Technologies, Limassol, Cyprus
e-mail: emariatos@avntechgroup.com

V. Karkaletsis et al. (eds.), *RADIO–Robots in Assisted Living*,
https://doi.org/10.1007/978-3-319-92330-7_7

transmission and processing; integrated and power-aware data collection, transmission, and processing; and an efficient and flexible architecture that can integrate heterogeneous health and comfort-related devices.

In the context of RADIO, the robot acts mainly as a mobile sensor platform that monitors and guides an elderly or disabled person throughout the entire day, using cameras and microphones as well as through direct access to the home automation infrastructure.

However, to achieve its mandate, the robot has to constantly know where the person is and to be able to move if the person moves to a new location or another room. While monitoring, the robot mechanical systems do not operate, thus saving battery life. But this is not enough; the power consumed by the main robot controller is significantly high, given that (even when not moving) a relatively powerful computing engine needs to be active. This holds true even during idle-time periods, e.g., when the person is sleeping or watching TV, as there is no way for the robot to know if and when the person intends to move. To reduce this idle-time power consumption wastage, as part of the RADIO project, a hardware (HW), FPGA-based implementation of event detection algorithms is set forward.

7.2 Data Collection and Processing

Assistive environments are typically implemented as smart homes or similar sensor networks that collect and analyze data related to mood and activities of daily life (ADL), as well as automatically providing notifications to caregivers when specific events are identified such as falls and similar emergencies. This is a well-studied subject with a rich literature and developed systems. One major line of research takes advantage of wearable sensors or sensors embedded in household items and appliances in order detect a wide range of ADLs [3–6]. Such approaches are not well aligned with the objective of developing a system that is unobtrusive by, among other features, also avoiding requirements on what the end-users should wear or use.

RADIO concept follows the line of research that uses computer vision and audio analysis to recognize interesting events. In fact, one of the main outcomes of the project is our analysis of the extent to which unobtrusive monitoring is adequate to meet stringent clinical requirements. To the best of our knowledge, the presented methodology is unique in assisted living environments; we do not assume as a goal the maximal detail and accuracy that state-of-the-art sensing hardware can achieve. Instead, we assume as a goal, the collection of the minimum amount of sensitive content and personal information, at the minimum obtrusion, that will allow medical personnel to make informed decisions.

Naturally, such a broadly defined goal needs to be refined to reflect the societal impact that RADIO aims to achieve: allowing elderly people with a mild cognitive impairment to maintain an independent life, at their own home, for longer than what is safely possible today. In order to have a guideline about what information is used by medical doctors to assess such conditions, the interRAI Long-Term Care Facilities Assessment System (interRAI LTCF) has been thoroughly analyzed. interRAI LTCF enables comprehensive, standardized evaluation of the needs, strengths, and preferences of persons receiving short-term post-acute care in skilled nursing facilities as well as persons living in chronic care and nursing home institutional settings. As a result, we have determined the mood and ADL recognition items that can be immediately and automatically extracted and those that appear to be outside the reach of the current state of the art.

Some characteristic examples include clothes change detection, where recognizing the end-result of having changed clothes [7] is sufficient while the detailed capture of all the motions performed in order to change clothes offers no medically relevant information. Similarly, depth camera data can be used to detect potentially dangerous activities [8] and food intake [9]. Moreover, acoustic processing can provide information about several ADLs, such as hygiene, washing, and walking [10]. Finally, the mood can be inferred from both visual and audio analysis [10–12].

These observations have led us to a design where the main data collection device is a mobile robot equipped with audio, visual, and depth camera. The mobility of the robotic platform is important for placing the sensors at positions that offer the maximum level of detail (e.g., full-face images for recognizing mood from facial expressions) without placing requirements of the end-user such as having to move in front of a sensor or having to use specific equipment. This choice, however, also introduces challenges due to the heterogeneity of the home automation and robotics infrastructures, as well as due to the low power consumption requirements necessary for having a mobile platform with sufficient battery autonomy.

7.3 The AAL Robot as a Heterogeneous Processing System

The RADIO robot is outfitted with two processing units: an Intel NUC which is responsible for controlling sensors and actuators and an Avnet PicoZed equipped with Xilinx Zynq-7000 all programmable System on Chip (APSoC) [13]. Additional devices include an Asus Xtion Pro camera and a Hokuyo laser scanner [14]. In general, there are two types of data processed in the system:

- *High throughput streaming data* created from continually receiving the output of a microphone (audio stream) or a camera (video stream)
- *Event or control-like data* of relatively small size, collected by sensors. Event/measurement data can also be the outcome of streaming data analysis, e.g., processing of video can lead to the generation of an "exit" event if the camera looks toward the door

External interfacing is achieved through RF networks with emphasis on low power and minimal usage of the RF spectrum. Adopted communication technologies are not suitable for conveying real-time streaming data like audio or video, leaving no other option, but to perform the processing of the multimedia workloads in the robot.

As mentioned, our AAL approach heavily relies on the acquisition and processing of audio and video streams for analyzing and recognizing activities of daily life (ADL) [7–9]. Recognizing the emotional status of patients and the identification of emergency situations, such as the detection of falls, are also of high importance [10–12]. As a result, the main processing engine(s) of robot are designed to operate as a power-efficient architecture for streaming data processing.

Apart from the FPGA fabric, the Xilinx PicoZed platform includes also an ARM Cortex A9 dual core processor (equipped with a Neon coprocessor) interfaced with programmable logic.

7.4 Fast and Energy-Efficient Data Processing

Figure 7.1 illustrates two different scenarios of positioning the robot processing elements and their interfaces. In both cases, the bulk of processing is indented to be performed on the FPGA platform. However, the two scenarios differ in the points where the sources of audio (microphone) and visual (camera) streams are located. The advantages and disadvantages of each scenario are analyzed in the rest of this section. In any case, the camera and audio data streams will be continuously monitored and when activity is detected the corresponding algorithms (which can analyze and recognize the activity) will be triggered. Depending on the specific combination of algorithms that get triggered, some or all computational tasks may be executed in the NUC, in the Zynq ARM processor, or accelerated with fixed logic or reconfigurable hardware components inserted in the FPGA reprogrammable logic.

In the second scenario depicted in Fig. 7.1, the camera and audio data streams, as provided through the NUC, will be continuously monitored by the processing elements of the FPGA platform. Therefore, a pipe that brings the streams down on the FPGA platform is implemented on the NUC using ROS channels. To avoid overloading the interface with unnecessary memory transfers, the ROS channels are constructed so that image and audio data is provided to the FPGA platform on a need-to-know basis. When the captured image data are transferred to the FPGA device (through ROS messages), the RAM which resides on board will be directly accessible from both the dual ARM core and the FPGA fabric (to minimize onboard memory transfers).

Figure 7.1 illustrates the streaming data flow through the robot processing elements and their interfaces. The camera and audio data streams are continuously monitored and when activity is detected the corresponding algorithms (which can analyze and recognize the activity) are triggered.

Depending on the specific combination of algorithms that gets triggered, some or all computational tasks may be executed in the (i) NUC, (ii) Zynq ARM processor, or (iii) accelerated by hardware components in the FPGA.

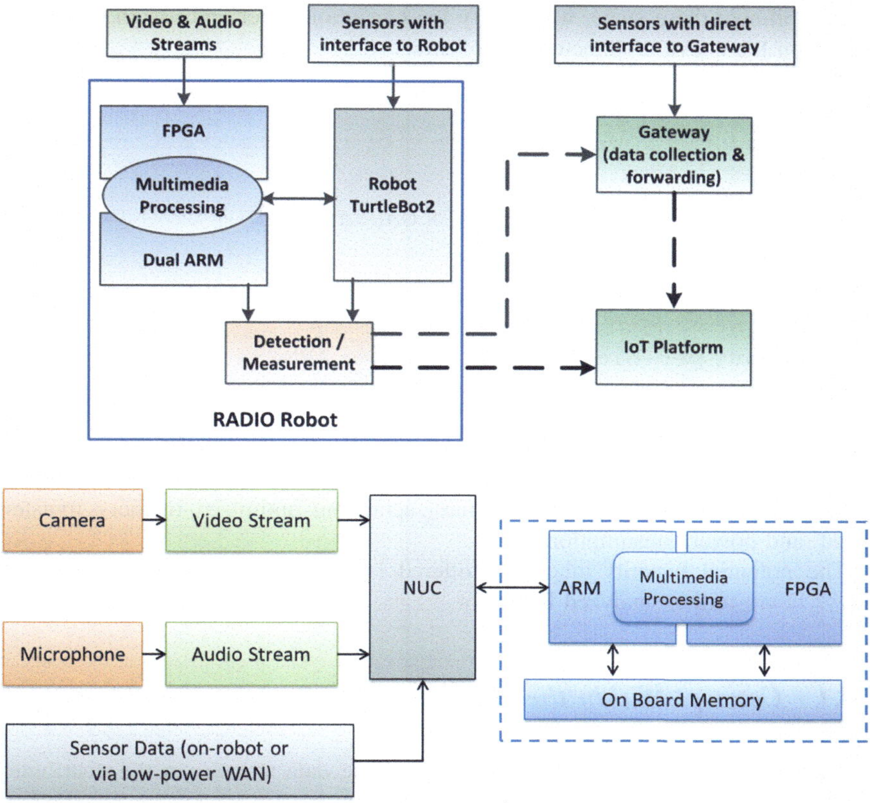

Fig. 7.1 Diagram illustrating two different scenarios of the data flow between the RADIO robot, gateway, and IoT platform

To provide a specific example of this concept, we describe here the implementation of the algorithm used in ADL "Measure time to get out of bed". Data processing with this algorithm consists of following (simplified) steps:

- `For each Frame`
  - `Store frame in RAM to be used as "previous" in next iteration`
  - `Split Frame in blocks of 9x9 pixels`
  - `Compare blocks with "previous frame" blocks to detect difference`
  - `Get bounding rectangle of all different blocks`
  - `Get centre of all different blocks`
  - `Check bounding rectangle and centre against the set limits`
  - `Report any events /findings`

To optimize these steps, we modify the execution order and assign to various blocks on the above architecture as follows:

- `For each frame (row 1 to row 469)`
  - `Get next 9 rows [Camera -> Video Stream -> NUC -> ARM]`
  - `For each row:`

    `Split in 9x9 blocks [ARM-> OnBoardRAM]`
    `For each block:`

    `Read 9x9 [OnBoardRAM-> FPGA]`
    `Compare and store "previous" [FPGA]`
    `Report per-block result [FPGA-> ARM]`
  - `Calculate Bounding and Centre [ARM]`
  - `Report to NUC [ARM-> NUC]`

This simplified example illustrates how a method can be adapted to fit the specific requirements of the architecture, achieving optimized memory transfer, speed, and power consumption.

The potential benefits inherently offered by the first scenario (illustrated in Fig. 7.1) are further analyzed below.

7.4.1 Concept Within the Distributed RADIO Environment

The need for fast and efficient processing of the data streams in the distributed RADIO environment comes from the need to be:

- *Responsive*: in some cases, the data collected on the robot and the measured/ detected quantities and events are correlated centrally with data from the smart home sensors or other sources. For example, detection of exiting the room can be correlated with a motion sensor mounted on the room walls
- *Energy Efficient*: as the robot relies on a battery, data processing should be limited to what is necessary and executed on the node yielding the lowest overall power consumption

To put this into perspective, an example state diagram of the robot is presented in Fig. 7.2.

In this diagram, we have two points (in green fonts) where entering is triggered by the smart-home infrastructure through getting the event from a motion sensor. There are also a number of states that involve heavy data processing and we have to ensure that this is either:

- very low power
  - time needed to stand up (gym)
  - measure walking speed (gym)

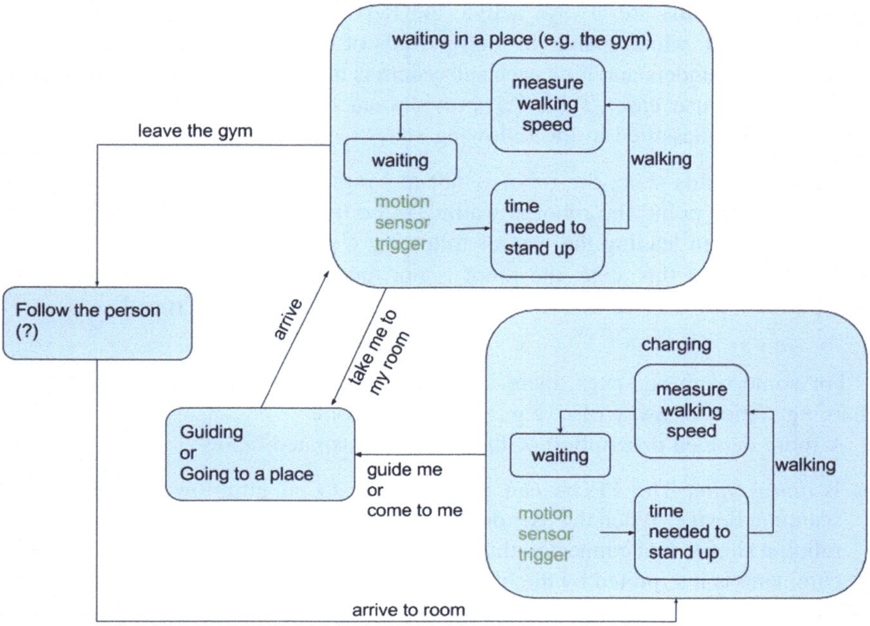

Fig. 7.2 State diagram highlighting different (power) modes

- follow the person
- guiding or going to a place

or

- executed when the robot is stationed on its charging station
  - time needed to stand up (in the room)
  - measure walking speed (in the room)

7.4.2 Modeling the Operational States of the AAL Robot

The RADIO robot is a unit which has many energy-hungry subsystems. These are

- Main processor to control robot movement (NUC)
- FPGA to accelerate ADL recognition methods
- Sensors, especially the image sensor (camera)
- Mechanical subsystem (motors)
- Wireless subsystem (network)

If all subsystems are always active, the RADIO robot needs to be recharged every few hours, which results in long periods of robot nonavailability. As a first step, we had to understand how each subsystem is used and if it, indeed, needs to be active at each use case. Table 7.1 provides an overview, assuming that robot activity can be classified in the following states:

- *Waiting*: at this state, the robot is not moving; neither is it processing sensor data. At this point, the robot is waiting to be triggered by some external event
- *Moving*: when leading the way or following a person
- *Monitoring*: at this state, the robot is not moving, but it is processing sensor input data in order to detect an ADL or understand patient's mood

For some of these states, there is a difference on whether the robot is on its charging station or away of it, e.g., in another room.

A more detailed description of the cases is illustrated below:

- *Waiting State*: The FPGA can connect only to an ultra-low power wireless scanning device. When the user or any other RADIO system wants to instruct the robot, it should first connect to this device, and send a handshake command. This command is interpreted by the FPGA. For example, it can be used to turn-on the CPU and perform a simple action. If more complex control is needed, e.g., a user request via the tablet GUI, the CPU will turn-on the network subsystem.
- *Monitoring/Away State*: At this state, the FPGA gets triggered by external events or continuously monitors live sensor signals. Only when some (external or sensor) activity occurs, the HW component in the FPGA will preprocess it and decide whether the CPU or/and the network subsystem has to be turned on.
- *Monitoring/Charging and Moving States*: At these states, we may not need to employ any on-demand approach for the CPU and/or the network. However, having the dedicated hardware components in the FPGA will allow some of the processing to be offloaded there, which also yields considerable energy benefits.

The energy consumed at each state by each subsystem is not the same. For example, the CPU while waiting can be clocked at a lower frequency, drastically reducing the required power. Also, sensors and FPGA can perform only basic data capture and processing when monitoring away from the charging dock and revert to full-power processing mode when this power is available.

Although a number of such techniques are used, their impact on power consumption is not drastic in all cases. To cope with this problem, our view is to

Table 7.1 Robot subsystem energy usage

State	CPU	FPGA	Sensor	Motors	Network
Waiting	Used	Not used	Not used	Not used	Used
Moving	Used	Used	Used	Used	Used
Monitoring/away	Used	Used	Used	Not used	Used
Monitoring/changing	Used	Used	Used	Not used	Used

Table 7.2 Energy profile by using HW accelerator

State	CPU	FPGA	Sensor	Motors	Network
Waiting	On demand	Used	Not used	Not used	On demand
Moving	Used	Used	Used	Used	Used
Monitoring/away	On demand	Used	Used	Not used	On demand
Monitoring/changing	Used	Used	Used	Not used	Used

develop dedicated hardware components that allow the robot to turn-off complete subsystems in some cases; turning them on only on demand and just for the short period when they are really needed. The goal is to have an improved energy profile. The results of this analysis are depicted in Table 7.2.

7.4.3 The Role of a Dedicated HW Component

A HW accelerator component is a specially designed circuit which is implemented in FPGA (for configurability and future upgradability) and is connected directly to the other subsystems. The component is processing signals from sensors, so that simple decisions on whether other subsystems have to be employed or not can be devised. Typically, this component is equipped with the following functionality:

- *Triggering mechanism*, which initiates sensor data capture and processing
- *Local memory*, which holds processed sensor data so that the main system RAM does not have to be used
- *Signal processing acceleration functions* in FPGA
- *Control interfaces* to turn-on and notify (or get notified by) other subsystems

In the context of RADIO, the dedicated HW components (see Sect. 7.6) are implemented in the programmable logic (PL) of the PicoZed APSoC using the Vivado HLS (High-level Synthesis) tool. The accelerators are optimized for performance and area and they proved flexible enough to perform their role: *early detection of a high possibility for an event so that SW-based processing can be invoked.*

7.5 Experimental Profiling and Results

7.5.1 Example ADL Use Cases

To prototype and experiment with the alternative approach discussed in this chapter, we selected a small number of ADLs as target use cases for the monitoring state of the robot. The selected ADL recognition methods must:

- Be able to be detected when the robot is not moving
- Have a significant part of preprocessing, which can be done on the FPGA

- Get triggered by some external signal or some very simple HW-only method
- Not rely on information exchanged over the WiFi or smart-home network

The selected methods will be the ones which detect:

- *The time that is needed by the patient to get out of bed.* This ADL is based on image processing algorithms that observe the patient while getting out of bed. The image processing algorithms can be parallelized availing themselves for the acceleration within the FPGA hardware. This algorithm divides the image into different regions. If the center of mass of moving pixels over succeeding images lies in one of these defined regions, an event is triggered. Thus, this algorithm is able to detect if a person is sleeping, awake but not going out of bed and awake and standing up.
- *Picking up medication cups.* The image processing methods used to detect this ADL benefit from the acceleration through the FPGA hardware as they rely on a complex algorithm.

The acceleration does not involve the complete method; but rather focuses on early detection of a high possibility for an event so that SW-based processing can be invoked. Specifically, for the above-mentioned ADLs:

- For the time-to-stand-up ADL, the hardware component will collect and calculate data from all regions, providing a trigger to software when a given activity threshold is crossed.
- For the cup-detection ADL, since this is manually triggered by the operator, hardware acceleration is not related to the recognition but to the stabilization and centering of the image. It has been observed through field trials that the robot can slightly move while waiting; a movement that might create false positives. An always running HW component will be monitoring such small movements and constantly re-center the view.

7.5.2 Optimizing for Power

In order to determine the SW–HW co-design of the FPGA-ARM system, extensive profiling of the image processing algorithms are needed (see Sect. 7.6). Generally, FPGAs provide high-performance when manipulating the images pixel-wise or in small blocks. This allows several hardware implementations with different degrees of parallelism. Each hardware design then must be evaluated within the overall RADIO framework in order to determine the best implementation.

At the first phase of the project, our work was allocated to have a working HW acceleration framework, and not to the specific optimization of each HW component. In a subsequent phase, we profiled three options, so that the expected benefits of various optimization approaches can be quantified, allowing to focus on these solutions that will yield the most benefits.

The three analyzed options—as described earlier—are as follows:

- *No-offloading*, all processing is performed on the robot's main processing unit (NUC)
- *Offload on embedded ARM core* of the FPGA (no HW acceleration)
- *Offload on dedicated low-level hardware blocks* in the FPGA (ARM core can be power down)

7.5.3 Profiling on Daily Activity Use Cases

To make a realistic profiling, we identified typical activity use cases with the help of nontechnical partners of the RADIO consortium. Each typical activity is depicted as a combination of five states for the robot subsystem:

- *Moving*, where the robot is actually moving and uses its motor, sensors, and camera
- *Monitoring*, where the robot is waiting for an event to be triggered by what it can see
- *Sensing*, where the robot is using its onboard sensors or communicates with smart home
- *Processing*, where heavy processing to analyze sensor and camera input is required
- *Idle*, where the robot is on but is doing nothing of the above

It is important to understand that a specific human activity (e.g., having lunch) will combine more than one of the above states (e.g., looking, sensing, and processing).

By accumulating the energy needs at each activity, we are able to extract the daily activity profile in terms of energy consumption as shown in Fig. 7.3. More specifically, the data presented in Fig. 7.3 are extracted by i) analyzing the daily activity patterns of the person(s) that is being monitored during the whole day

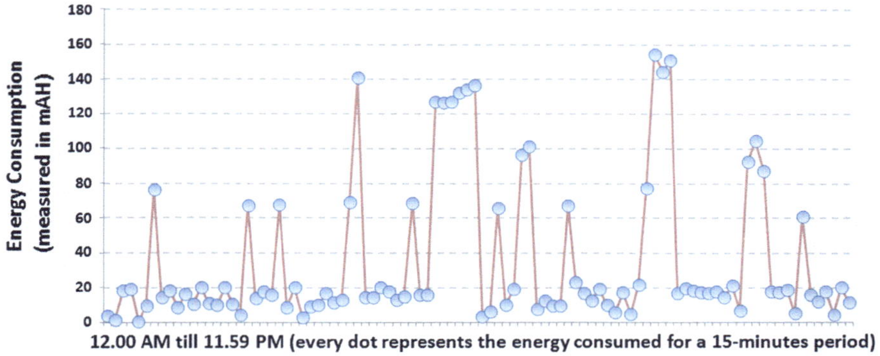

Fig. 7.3 Daily activity profile

(24 h) in their domestic environment and ii) conducting live measurements to calculate the energy consumed in each discrete phase of the robot (consequently in each activity of the target person) assuming that all data processing is performed in NUC. Finally, we should mention that the daily activity patterns were collected by personal caregivers during the third pilot phase of the RADIO project and represent the (averaged) activity patterns of three persons.

7.5.4 Power-Saving Results

The three options analyzed in the previous section are then tested on the profile illustrated in Fig. 7.3. Our target is to reveal the potential for maximizing battery life in terms of reducing the required re-charges during the day; in other words, to increase the autonomy of the AAL robot by using specialized hardware accelerators. The target areas are the points located in the lower part of Fig. 7.3 (juxtaposed the x-axis). These points correspond to the cases in which the robot is either in the sensing or idle state waiting for an event to occur.

To this end, we performed a battery load calculation and our results are presented in Fig. 7.4. The vertical axis in Fig. 7.4 shows the battery level of the robotic platform, whereas the horizontal axis represents the day-time period (every dot point in the lines is associated to a battery-level measurement taken every 15 minutes). There are three lines in the figure corresponding to the three studied offloading policies: (i) no offload (green line), (ii) offload on the embedded ARM core of the FPGA platform (blue line), and (iii) offload on dedicated low-level hardware blocks in the FPGA (red line). Finally, in all cases, the sharp ramp-ups indicate the battery charging periods.

As Fig. 7.4 indicates, our offloading policies are able to significantly increase the autonomy of the robot. In our setup, the time required to charge the battery (from depletion to full capacity) is a 2-h period. As a result, in the "no-offloading" case, for a time-window equal to 4 h, the robot is not able to operate, thus it cannot follow the person to another room or most importantly it might miss capturing important data that are relevant to a critical situation or emergency. In addition, the charging periods coincide with periods of increased activity (as indicated by the results presented in Fig. 7.3). On the contrary, our offloading policies (e.g., when the wake-up decision logic is implemented in the FPGA) manage to reduce the number of the required charges to one and to actually move the charging period to a time slot of reduced activity.

7.6 Accelerating Image Processing Algorithms

The algorithm for monitoring the state of the patient is based on the center of gravity calculation and can be divided into 4 to 5 parts, depending on whether markups are activated or not. Figure 7.5 shows the general functionality of the algorithm as schematic and as pseudocode.

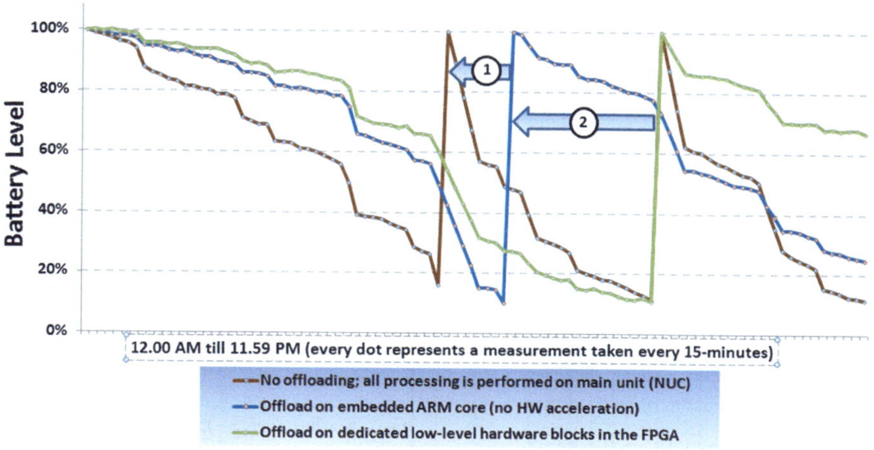

Fig. 7.4 Run-time depletion of robot battery and number of required charges for the three studied offloading policies

1. *Reading of the most recent image frame*: The image data is provided by the Asus Xtion Pro camera of the RADIO robot platform. The image data is sent via USB directly to the NUC which publishes the received frames via its robot operating system to the Avnet PicoZed where it is processed. The image frame is then read by the software and saved to a 3-dimensional array. The first two dimensions indicate the pixels positions whereas the third dimension stores the color values of the RGB color channel. Each color is coded with 8 bit, resulting in the 24-bit color payload. Given that the Asus Xtion Pro camera provides images with the size of 640×480 pixels, the resulting array size is $640 \times 480.3 = 921{,}600$ or 900 KiB.
2. *Detection of movement*: The algorithm loads subsequent frames and compares both image frames with each other in order to detect changes or movement within the two image frames. In order to reduce the impact of small movements of the camera or image noise, the comparison does not only take place on the subtracted image, but rather also on blocks of pixels. Within these blocks, the mean value of all subtracted color channels is calculated. If this value exceeds a certain threshold, the respective block is flagged as active to show that a change has occurred. While the person is moving out of the bed, the pixel blocks that detect movement are highlighted in red.
3. *Calculation of center of gravity*: After all blocks have either been detected as active or inactive, the center of gravity can be calculated. In this case, the center of gravity is calculated through the mean value of the positions of all active blocks. Because the active blocks are positioned in the middle of the image and in the lower right corner of the image, the center of gravity lies directly in the between of the detected hotspots of movement.

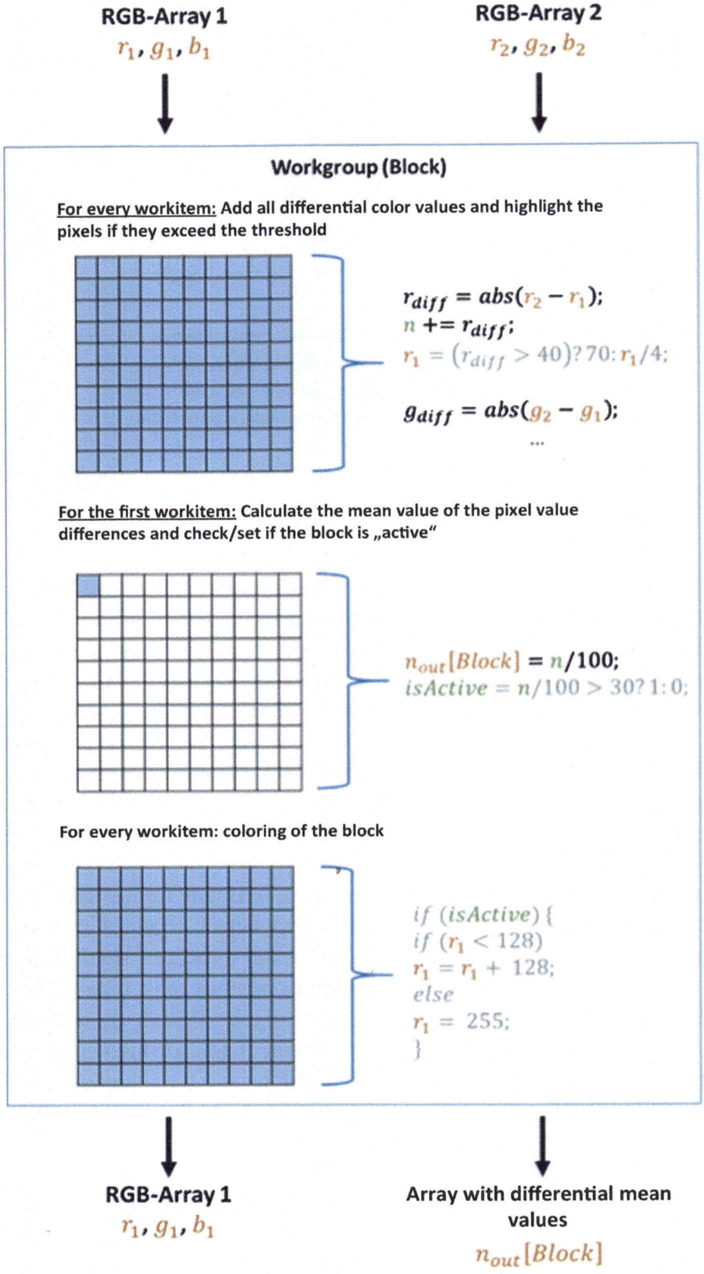

Fig. 7.5 Schematic view of the kernel design annotated with pseudocode

4. *Evaluation of center of gravity*: Now that the position of the center of gravity has been determined, its position needs to be analyzed and interpreted. If the y-coordinate of the center of gravity exceeds a certain threshold, the algorithm assumes that the observed person has gotten out of bed. Several of these thresholds exist.
5. *Drawing markups*: In order to optimize and debug the algorithm, markups can be drawn into the image. When drawing markups, all color values which differ more than the value 40 compared to the prior frame are set to 70. If the pixels differ less than 40, the color values are quartered. Additionally, the pixel within an active block will be colored red. This is done by adding the value 128 to the red channel. This calculation is saturated, meaning that the resulting value never exceeds 255.

7.6.1 Profiling Results

In order to optimally accelerate the image processing algorithm with programmable hardware, the computer-intensive components need to be identified. This is done with the help of profiling. The PicoZed is a System on Chip with a dual core ARM Cortex A9 processor and integrated programmable hardware. The image processing algorithm is first executed on the ARM processor. There, the performance of the algorithm is determined and the potential hardware-accelerated components are identified. From the software side, the algorithm consists of several sub-blocks which are further analyzed during the profiling. These are described in Table 7.3.

For each profiling run, the algorithm is executed 20 times in order to mitigate the impact of outliers. The used profiler is gprof and the results are presented in Fig. 7.6 for the algorithm with markups and in Fig. 7.7 for the algorithm without markups.

As can be seen in both figures, the algorithm spends most of the total processing time in the *checkBoxes* function. In the case of activated markups, the amount is 61.70% and 51.20% without activated markups. Because the *copyToImageData* function is only required for debug purposes, this function will not be implemented in the final algorithm design. Therefore, the timing value for this function is ignored. In the case of activated markups, all the data required for the *annotateBoxes* function is generated by the *checkBoxes* function. Because both functions are executed sequentially, it is possible to generate hardware accelerators for both functions.

7.6.2 Hardware Accelerator Design

In order to efficiently switch between the algorithm with and without markup functionality, two OpenCL kernels are designed. This enables an efficient

Table 7.3 Subblock of the algorithm

Profiled functions of the algorithm	
Function name	Task
copyToRGB	Copy the received image data to a 3-dimensional array
Checkboxes	Calculate the mean value of the color value differences over the last 2 frames and indicate the active blocks
annotateBoxes	If markups are activated, indicate the pixel changes and highlight the active blocks
process_function	Calculates the center of gravity and determines its position. This is the function that calls *checkBoxes* and *annotateBoxes*
copyToImageData	Copy the processed image data from the 3-dimensional array to a ROS compatible array for debug purposes

```
  %   cumulative   self              self     total
 time   seconds   seconds    calls  ms/call  ms/call  name
61.70      2.32     2.32    61440     0.04     0.04  checkBoxes
17.02      2.96     0.64       20    32.00    32.00  copyToImageData
16.49      3.58     0.62       20    31.00    31.00  copyToRGB
 3.72      3.72     0.14    13199     0.01     0.01  annotateBoxes
 1.06      3.76     0.04       20     2.00   125.00  process_function
```

Fig. 7.6 Profiling results of the algorithm with activated markups

implementation of only one query in order to determine which kernel version will be executed. OpenCL kernels consist of workgroups and workitems. In this case, a workgroup stands for one-pixel block and a workitem stands for one pixel. The designed kernel will then be called $640 \times 480 = 307{,}200$ times for each pixel pair. The first step is to calculate the difference of all color values of each pixel pair in a workgroup. If the differential value exceeds the value 40, the pixel value is set to 70, otherwise, the value is divided by 4. As soon as each workitem of a workgroup completes the differential calculation, the first workitem of the workgroup will calculate the mean value of all workitems. The mean value is then saved to an external array which is accessible by the CPU for further processing. If the mean value exceeds the threshold value of 30, the block will be highlighted in red. Figure 7.8 shows the kernel implementation as schematic and as pseudocode.

The initial version of the OpenCL code can be generated with 100 MHz. Figure 7.9 shows the resource requirements of the initial hardware version. This core is compared to a software implementation on the dual core processor of the PicoZed. The execution time of the algorithm on software takes approximately 17,547 μs. The generated hardware requires 88404 μs, meaning the hardware accelerator requires 88404 μs or (at 100 MHz) 8840400 cycles to execute the algorithm. This results in a speedup of 0.2. In order to achieve an accelerator which actually accelerates the image processing algorithm, further optimization steps have to be executed.

% time	cumulative seconds	self seconds	calls	self ms/call	total ms/call	name
51.29	1.39	1.39	61440	0.02	0.02	checkBoxes
26.57	2.11	0.72	20	36.00	36.00	copyToImageData
21.03	2.68	0.57	20	28.50	28.50	copyToRGB
0.74	2.70	0.02	20	1.00	70.50	process function

Fig. 7.7 Profiling results of the algorithm without activated markups

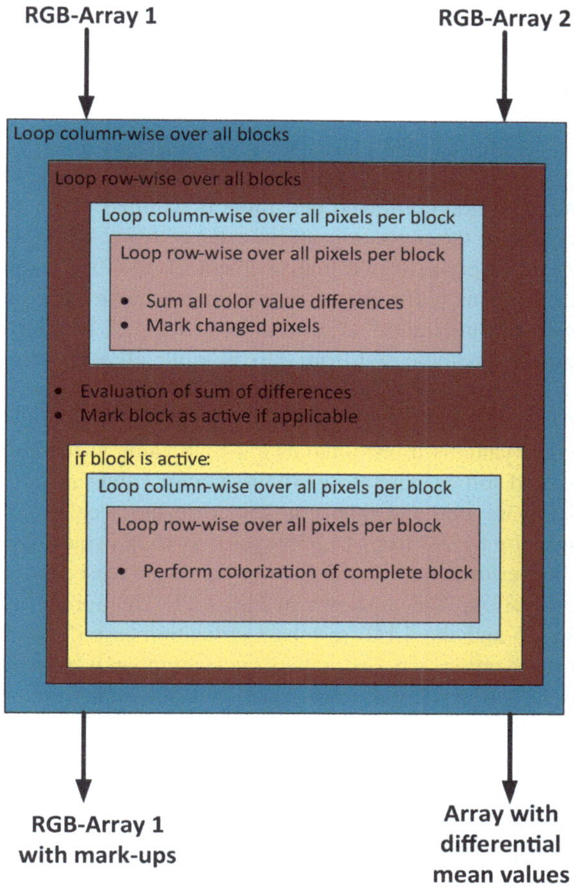

Fig. 7.8 Depiction of the implemented algorithm

The first optimization step is to efficiently let the accelerator read the image data from the DDR memory. This is done with the command *async_work_group_copy*. This command transmits a user-defined number of sequential bytes from memory via a burst mode to the accelerator. The transmission of one frame is executed stepwise in order to reduce the resource usage of the BRAM on the programmable

Fig. 7.9 Resource utilization of the initial OpenCL kernel

Name	BRAM_18K	DSP48E	FF	LUT
DSP	-	-	-	-
Expression	-	-	0	1827
FIFO	-	-	-	-
Instance	2	4	662	812
Memory	-	-	-	-
Multiplexer	-	-	-	2599
Register	-	-	2160	-
Total	2	4	2822	5238
Available	280	220	106400	53200
Utilization (%)	~0	1	2	9

hardware. Because one image always lies sequentially in memory, only one transmission command per frame is required. After this step, the estimate cycles to complete the algorithm are in a range from 4,729,607 to 5,712,647 cycles, which means a performance improvement of 36–46% compared to the initial implementation. This performance improvement, however, comes at the cost of an increased resource utilization as can be seen in Fig. 7.10. Here, the number of used BRAM blocks has increased from 2 to 74 while all other resources remain almost constant.

Because the number of required BRAMs is very high, the memory requirements of the accelerator are reduced in the second optimization step. Currently, every color value is transmitted as a 4-byte value to the BRAMs although a 1-byte value would suffice. Therefore, all three color values are stored in one 4-byte value on the software side and then transmitted to the accelerator. This reduces the data transmission by 2/3 from 14,535 cycles to 4935 cycles. By performing this optimization, the performance of the accelerator is increased while also reducing the resource utilization. This is shown in Fig. 7.11. The number of BRAMs is reduced from 74 to 42 and the LUT resource utilization is reduced by 2% compared to the first optimization. The estimated cycle number is also further reduced to 2,272,007–2,947,847 cycles which is a performance improvement of 52% compared to the first optimization step.

Since image processing algorithms perform many operations on each pixel individually, these operations are executed in a loop. These loops can be parallelized on hardware. Parallelizing a loop can be done through loop pipelining or through loop unrolling. While loop pipelining reuses the already available components for parallelization, loop unrolling requires separate resources in order to increase the degree of parallelism. Therefore, loop pipelining requires less additional resources than loop unrolling. The algorithm has 5 loops that can benefit from either loop unrolling or loop pipelining, see Fig. 7.5. In the case of this algorithm, no performance difference is detected when using loop unrolling compared to loop pipelining. Because loop pipelining requires less hardware resources, loop pipelining is used for 2 of the 5 loops. In the other 3 loops, no performance improvement was measured when employing pipelining or unrolling techniques.

Fig. 7.10 Resource utilization of the OpenCL kernel after optimizing the data access

Name	BRAM_18K	DSP48E	FF	LUT
DSP	-	-	-	-
Expression	-	-	0	1591
FIFO	-	-	-	-
Instance	2	4	662	812
Memory	72	-	0	0
Multiplexer	-	-	-	1340
Register	-	-	1786	150
Total	74	4	2448	3893
Available	280	220	106400	53200
Utilization (%)	26	1	2	7

Fig. 7.11 Resource utilization of the OpenCL kernel after optimizing memory requirements

Name	BRAM_18K	DSP48E	FF	LUT
DSP	-	-	-	-
Expression	-	-	0	691
FIFO	-	-	-	-
Instance	2	4	662	812
Memory	40	-	0	0
Multiplexer	-	-	-	1245
Register	-	-	1383	140
Total	42	4	2045	2888
Available	280	220	106400	53200
Utilization (%)	15	1	1	5

Figure 7.12 shows the resource utilization when employing loop pipelining for the algorithm. Through loop pipelining, the resource requirements of the BRAMs are reduced even further from 42 to 38. The number of DSP blocks is also reduced from 4 to 1 and the FFs are slightly increased as well as the LUT resource usage. This optimization further increased the performance compared to the last optimization step, leading to the cycle number of 1,273,607–1,586,951 which is an acceleration of 44–46%.

After these three optimization steps, the accelerator is again compared to the software implementation of the algorithm.

7.6.3 Evaluation

In order to evaluate the performance of the accelerator on the real hardware, the accelerator must first be implemented on the PicoZed platform. This is done with

Fig. 7.12 Resource utilization of the OpenCL kernel after optimizing loop executions

Name	BRAM_18K	DSP48E	FF	LUT
DSP	-	1	-	-
Expression	-	-	0	2142
FIFO	-	-	-	-
Instance	2	-	662	812
Memory	36	-	0	0
Multiplexer	-	-	-	1344
Register	-	-	1927	140
Total	38	1	2589	4438
Available	280	220	106400	53200
Utilization (%)	13	~0	2	8

Table 7.4 Energy profile by using HW accelerator

Execution times and speedup compared to the software implementation		
Measurement platform	Execution time (μs)	Speedup
Software (ARM)	17,547	1
Initial implementation	88,404	0.2
First optimization	48,687	0.37
Second optimization	23,401	0.75
Third optimization	13,290	1.32

the Vivado tool provided by Xilinx. The accelerator must be connected to the processing system in order to receive the image data from the DDR memory. Table 7.4 shows the execution times of the different versions. For all implementations, the clock frequency of 100 MHz is used. The ARM processor is running at 666 MHz. It can be seen that the initial and up until the second optimization hardware version, the software version outperforms the hardware implementation. These changes in the third optimization where the hardware implementation reaches a speedup of 1.32 compared to the software version. All hardware implementations can further increase their performance compared to the software implementation by increasing the clock frequency.

7.7 Summary

This chapter presents the system-level approach followed in the RADIO project targeting to increase the autonomy (measured in terms of battery charges) of the robotic platform in AAL environments. The proposed approach is benchmarked in experimental conditions via use case profiling and it is driven by the daily activity patterns of the target elderly or disable people. The daily activity patterns were collected by caregivers personnel during the third pilot phase of the RADIO project.

As part of this, a general behavior concept is presented in this book chapter, which allows the robot to switch between extremely low power states and active state when necessary based on user behavior.

Special emphasis is given to fully utilize the robot processing units in the most efficient manner (APSoC with an ARM-based processing system and an FPGA programmable logic). This enables the robot to perform computation-intensive tasks very efficiently and very fast. However, in order to extract the most performance out of these processing units, all tasks that need to be executed by the robot platform have to be analyzed and scheduled accordingly on the processing system or on the programmable logic.

Finally, the FPGA implementation of an image processing algorithm for monitoring the state of the patient is also presented. All aspects of the implementation are provided, while detailed statistics (FPGA resource utilization and speedup) related to the efficiency of the FPGA acceleration are also offered. The design of the accelerator followed the hardware–software partitioning approach and it is based on the HLS (high-level synthesis) paradigm in order to reduce the programmability and development effort.

References

1. EU project RADIO. http://www.radio-project.eu.
2. Antonopoulos, C. P., Keramidas, G., Voros, N. S., Hübner, M., Göhringer, D., Dagioglou, M., et al. (2015). Robots in assisted living environments as an unobtrusive, efficient, reliable and modular solution for independent ageing: The RADIO Perspective. In *Proceedings of International Sympocium in Applied Reconfigurable Computing.*
3. Matic, A., Mehta, P., Rehg, J. M., Osmani, V., & Mayora, O. (2012). Monitoring dressing activity failures through RFID and video. *Methods of Information in Medicine.*
4. Philipose, M., Fishkin, K. P., Perkowitz, M., Patterson, D. J., Fox, D., Kautz, H., et al. (2004). Inferring activities from interactions with objects. *Pervasive Computing.*
5. Cook, D. J., & Schmitter-Edgecombe, M. (2009). Assessing the quality of activities in a smart environment. *Methods of Information in Medicine.*
6. Dalton, A. F., Morgan, F., & Olaighin, G. (2008). A preliminary study of using wireless kinematic sensors to identify basic activities of daily living. In *Proceedings of International Conference on Engineering in Medicine and Biology Society.*
7. Sgouropoulos, D., Giannakopoulos, T., Petridis, S., Perantonis, S., & Korakis, A. (2014). Clothes change detection using the Kinect sensor. In *Proceedings of International Conference on Signal Processing and Multimedia Applications.*
8. Zhang, C., & Tian, Y. (2012). RGB-D camera-based daily living activity recognition. *Journal of Computer Vision and Image Processing.*
9. Hondori, H. M., Khademi, M., & Lopes, C. V. (2012). Monitoring intake gestures using sensor fusion (microsoft kinect and inertial sensors) for smart home telerehab setting. In *Proceedings of Annual Healthcare Innovation Conference.*
10. Vacher, M., Fleury, A., Portet, F., Serignat, J.-F., & Noury, N. (2010). Complete sound and speech recognition system for health smart homes: Application to the recognition of activities of daily living. *New Developments in Biomedical Engineering.*
11. Koolagudi, S., & Rao, K. S. (2012). Emotion recognition from speech: A review. *Journal of Speech Technology.*

12. Zeng, Z., Pantic, M., Roisman, G. I., & Huang, T. S. (2009). A survey of affect recognition methods: Audio, visual, and spontaneous expressions. T*ransactions on Pattern Analysis and Machine Intelligence*.
13. Xilinx Inc. Zynq-7000 All Programmable SoC Overview, 2015.
14. TurtleBot2 Robot Development Kit. http://www.turtlebot.com.

Chapter 8
Designing User Interfaces for the Elderly

Maria Rigou, Spiros Sirmakessis, Raquel Ventura, Alberto Fernández, Christos P. Antonopoulos and Nikolaos Voros

8.1 Introduction: GUI Design Requirements for the Elderly

The world population is steadily and rapidly aging. According to a recent United Nations report [1], "*in 2017 the global population aged 60 years or over numbered 962 million*," which is more than twice as large as in 1980. This is a phenomenon that is more intense in developed countries with Europe and Northern America having the highest percentages of aging population with more than one person in five aged 60 or over. With all estimations converging to the assumption that this increase in aging percentages will continue in the coming years, governments and policy makers must take adequate measures to handle the induced

M. Rigou (✉)
Department of Computer Engineering and Informatics, University of Patras, Patras, Greece
e-mail: rigou@ceid.upatras.gr

S. Sirmakessis
Computer and Informatics Engineering Department, Technological Educational Institution of Western Greece, Patras, Greece
e-mail: syrma@teiwest.gr

R. Ventura · A. Fernández
Sensing & Control Systems S.L., Barcelona, Spain
e-mail: raquel.ventura@sensingcontrol.com

A. Fernández
e-mail: alberto.fernandez@sensingcontrol.com

C. P. Antonopoulos · N. Voros
Embedded System Design and Application Lab, Computer and Informatics Engineering Department, Technological Educational Institution of Western Greece, Patras, Greece
e-mail: cantonopoulos@teiwest.gr

N. Voros
e-mail: voros@teiwest.gr

V. Karkaletsis et al. (eds.), *RADIO–Robots in Assisted Living*,
https://doi.org/10.1007/978-3-319-92330-7_8

implications for nearly all sectors of society (labor and financial markets, demand for goods and services such as housing, transportation, and social protection). Software applications and device design could not remain unaffected by this aging phenomenon. In fact, research in the field of interaction design and ergonomics has been quite active and has provided guidelines and good practices to guide developers in delivering products and services that can be used by elderly users [2–9]. For defining design guidelines and being able to assess an application/device suitability for elderly users it is necessary to consider the characteristics (i.e., skills and limitations) of those users concerning software and device usage.

The usability of an application describes the degree to which the indented users can access the provided functionality and use it effectively. According to Nielsen [10], usability can be expressed and evaluated in terms of five attributes of a software application:

- **Learnability**: should be easy to learn the way to use it.
- **Efficiency**: should allow users to achieve their tasks within a reasonable amount of time.
- **Memorability**: should be easy to remember how to use it even after a long period of non-usage.
- **Errors**: should prevent user errors and provide recovery mechanisms in case errors occur.
- **Satisfaction**: should be pleasant to use (minimized frustration, fatigue, or dissatisfaction induced).

Age-related impairments influence the way people use computer systems and handheld mobile devices, the five attributes of usable applications named above must be considered from a stricter point of view. For instance, an application that is easy to learn for a teenager or a 35-year-old person may not be easy enough to learn for a 68-year old. Or, an on-screen target may have sufficient size and spacing to tap for a 40-year old but may result in numerous unsuccessful attempts for a 70-year old. Physical and cognitive restrictions/limitations which often occur with advancing age, influence usability aspects by imposing additional requirements. GUI and interaction designers define additional or more strict guidelines when a software addresses the elderly, based on the kind of physical and cognitive limitations affecting software usage for this target population. These limitations include reduced visual ability, hearing loss, psychomotor impairments, loss of fine motor control, attention-related factors, learning, and memory impairments [11].

According to research, touch-screen devices reduce cognitive and coordination demands [12] and are preferred for elder users [13] but the intuitiveness of using them does not guarantee that older users will manage to learn how to interact with them or that there will be no inadvertent activation due to difficulties in tasks that require precision [3]. Current touch-screen devices allow for single-touch or multi-touch interaction [14] depending on whether interaction is based on one point of contact (e.g., a finger) or on multiple simultaneous touch points [15] (e.g., fingers of a single hand or both hands using recognizable gestures). [3] after analyzing 568 different gestures provided the following classification of gestures on a multi-touch device:

- *Indexical gestures*: The user positions the finger on a certain screen object or region (e.g., a simple tap)
- *Manipulative gestures*: The user manipulates screen objects or regions using movement patterns such as repeated tapping, long presses, dragging movements, swift swipe or flick movements, spreading or pinching movements, encircling or boxing screen objects, etc.
- *Alphanumeric gestures*: The user draws one or more letters or numbers with the finger on the screen.
- *Iconic gestures*: The user draws real world objects (e.g., arrows, crosses, houses, magnifying glass, ear, loudspeaker, etc.).
- *Symbolic gestures*: A sign that is neither an iconic object representation nor an alphanumeric character (e.g. a minus, plus, bracket, question mark, etc.)
- *Combined*: a gesture that combines separate parts that belong to other gesture categories.

On multi-touch devices and depending on the operating system a large number of gestures may be supported to offer fast execution of numerous tasks. This approach offers tremendous speed and productivity to young, technology-savvy and experienced users but may cause confusion and hindrance to seniors. Guidelines elaborated specifically for software applications executed on a multi-touch device and targeted to elderly users should be thoroughly examined to ensure usability for the intended user population.

8.2 GUI Design Good Practices

Apart from the five aforementioned attributes of a usable software application, evaluations often use a set of heuristic rules as guidance through system examination. One of the most widely used set of heuristics was proposed by Nielsen and Molich [16] and revised by Nielsen [10]. According to it, a usable system should provide/support: (1) Visibility of system status, (2) Convergence between system and the real world, (3) User control and freedom, (4) Consistency and standards (5) Error prevention (6) Recognition rather than recall (7) Flexibility and efficiency of use, (8) Aesthetic and minimalist design, (9) Help users recognize, diagnose and recover from errors, and (10) Help and documentation.

Those heuristics provide a general guide for the evaluator and usually they are further elaborated and analyzed to a set of more tangible guidelines depending on the nature of the application and the characteristics of its intended users. For instance, for applications for elderly users, consistency is a central heuristic due to the characteristics of aging users. Every application requires a certain amount of training to memorize how to use it (and it is assessed as learnability level) and this knowledge is called “procedural memory” [17]. Though older adults have more difficulties in learning new procedures and a consistent design guarantees that less new processes or actions have to be learned. In addition, since for elderly users the knowledge of already internalized activities (e.g., the knowledge how to multiply two numbers) stays intact, designers should make use of standards and widely used conventions as much as possible.

In the case of the RADIO robot UI they were combined with a set of 58 specific guidelines for elderly users of tablet devices, proposed by Blendinger [18], in an effort to consider the full range of limitations imposed to users by aging. The guidelines are classified into seven groups that refer to different aspects of user interaction with a multi-touch device:

- **Design** refers to visual elements and the overall stimuli (colors, contrast, typeface, images, etc.) an interface generates for its users. Elderly users experience vision decline that causes changes in visual acuity or color perception.
- **Layout** concerns the relative positioning and sizing of screen contents (buttons, text block, etc.). Elderly users face motor and visual impairments that make reading text and reaching targets on touch screens more difficult. Another issue is where and how to display information on screen, as visual impairments, decline in attention and working memory may influence the perception of content [19]. Moreover, the navigation a user has to follow to reach the intended information/action should be designed in a way that visual clues are evident to the elderly user and are understood as such, avoiding confusion caused by deep hierarchies and large number of options.
- **Language and Wording** refers to all textual contents displayed to the user in terms of phrasing. Simple and positively phrased language is the key to make an application understandable and in the case of elderly users who tend to be more cautious in clicking on links or buttons [20–22] feel uncomfortable in trying new things [22] and need reassurance when using computer devices and software.
- **Icons, Graphics and Multimedia**. Icons and graphics convey information about functionality without using words. This is based on the assumption that a familiar visual representation is self-explanatory and is more easily and quickly understood by users, especially elderly users that take longer to read labels and textual descriptions. Nevertheless, it is safer to accompany icons with labels in case the user needs reassurance that understood correctly the icon. When there is also verbal information to be communicated to the user it is required to avoid frequencies above 4000 Hz as the frequency spectrum that can be perceived diminishes with age. A slower speech rate as well as avoiding background noises or music furthermore supports older people [19, 20].
- **Interaction** in the case of multi-touch devices for elderly users, concerns mainly two factors; whether a gesture on a touch screen is too complicated to execute (due to motor impairments) and whether it is hard to memorize a gesture and associate it with an action (due to cognitive difficulties that come with age). The second factor is more frequent the cause of an error than insufficient manual

dexterity to perform the gesture [3]. Also the lack of visual clues for typical gestures (e.g., zooming with a pinch gesture) demands from the user to learn and recall it but this may be a serious obstacle for the elderly [23]. Providing visual clues, adequate instructions and training may drastically help. In addition and in terms of gesture execution simplicity, indexical and manipulative gestures are typically recommended and overall rated to be more suitable than symbolic or iconic gestures [3, 24, 25]. Apart from gestures, interaction guidelines concern data entry, a task that should be kept to a minimum due to motor impairments (diminishing pointing accuracy) that lead to slow input speed and cognitive impairments (low-working memory capacity) thus requiring more concentration [17, 19]. Data entry should be supported (e.g., by offering correction options [13] or using a set of prepared phrases) and the on-screen keyboard should have larger buttons and adequate spacing for preventing accidental typing. Feedback is another major part of interaction as users always expect some kind of response from the system that their previous action had any effect and what was it (in order to determine if it was successful or not). On touch devices feedback is possible through visual, tactile, or auditory signals as well as through a combination of them. To ensure that especially older users can sense and interpret feedback properly, several age-related sensory changes have to be considered (e.g., low vision and hearing capabilities).

- **User Support and Training** is the 10th Nielsen heuristic and its value is crucial in the case of elderly users. All users must be provided with assistance on using a new application but the needs of aging users are much bigger as they may suffer from cognitive changes, have doubts about their ability to learn or tend to avoid getting into new learning situations [17]. Due to decline in cognitive abilities older users should not be provided with many alternative sources of help but the few (or the single) option that is offered should be sufficient, accessible, and comprehensible. Another recommended approach is to gradually introduce advanced features in order to prevent cognitive overload [26].
- **Personalization** refers to providing customization options that allow the user to fit certain application features to personal skills and limitations. This is very important in the case of older users as not all the elderly face the same declines at the same degree, nor do they occur at a specific age. This is the reason why the individual capabilities vary much more among older than younger age groups [17]. Customizable features may include font size, target size or annotation, type of feedback (visual and/or tactile and/or audio and their tuning), data entry mode (on-screen keyboard or physical), degree of functionality offered (a subset of features to fit novices or a full-feature range to fit experts). Attention should be given so that the personalization options are not so many or complicated that the elderly user cannot set appropriate values and make the correct selections.

8.3 enControl GUI Design

This section describes the graphical user interface for controlling and managing the home environment using a web-based application in the context of RADIO project.

8.3.1 Login to the Service

The web-based application can be opened by using different types of web browsers (Internet Explorer, Google Chrome, Mozilla Firefox, etc.) through the address line, type: http://domainofserviceprovider/Account/Login. A username and a password are supplied with the welcome to the service email that is sent when the account is activated (Fig. 8.1).

8.3.2 User Settings

To access the personal account area, a sub-menu allows you to access the *Settings, Help and Log off* sections (Fig. 8.2).

The *Settings* window allows you to change your password and language. You can also choose Celsius or Fahrenheit along with your Time Zone. Next, you can add the phone number and the email address in which you want to receive the notifications. By clicking on *Advanced* button you could choose the type of notifications you want to receive according to its section. Also you can set your default installation and the section you want to first watch in the platform (Fig. 8.3).

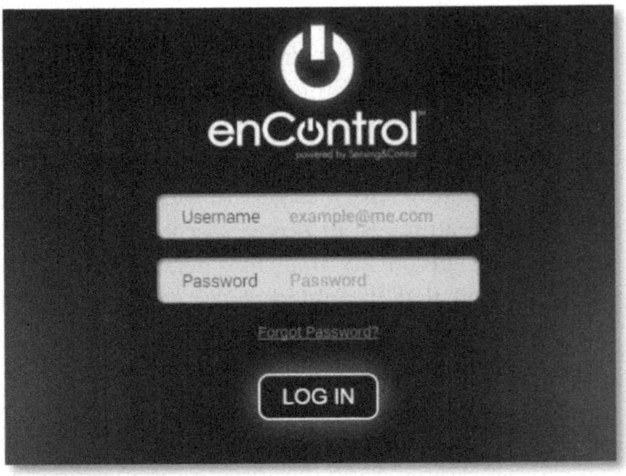

Fig. 8.1 Login screen

Fig. 8.2 User setting link

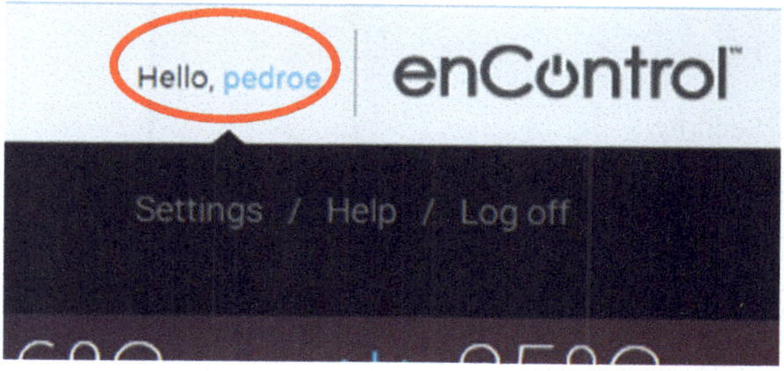

Tick which type of notification you want to receive for each functionality. Mail column will send you an email. Push will send a notifications to your mobile phone via enControl APP (if installed). If you select last column, neither mail/push nor event will be register in your inbox. With no column selected, you will get events in your inbox only. Remember to press save before you leave this view, otherwise changes will not take effect (Fig. 8.4).

For help using your enControl service, hover your mouse over the right-hand side of the menu bar and click *Help*. You will be redirected to www.encontrol.io/support-area. Where your will find a list of frequently asked questions to quickly help you with any problems you may have. Have a question that is not on the list?

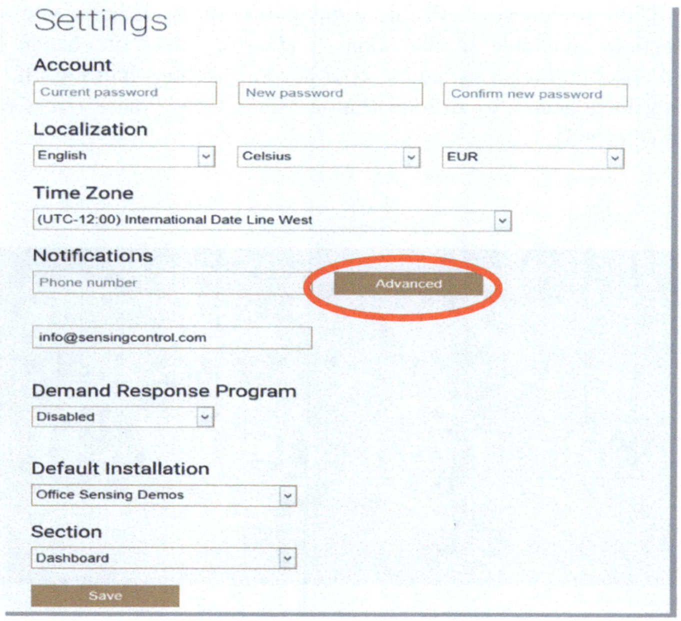

Fig. 8.3 User setting options

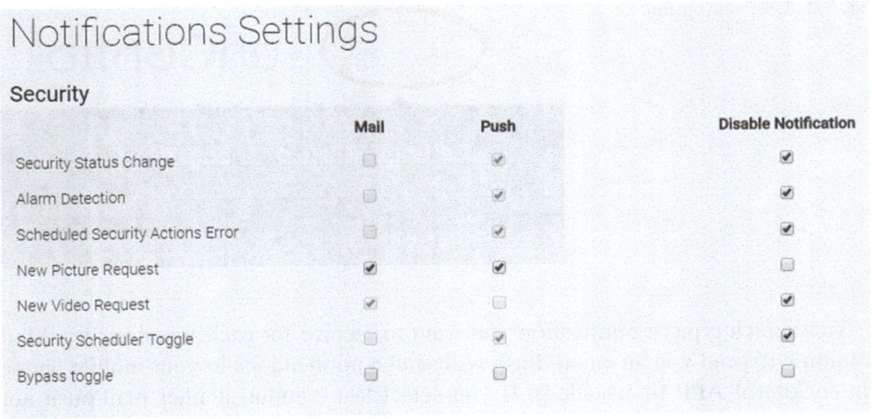

Fig. 8.4 Notification settings options

Just jump to ticket support areas at https://encontrol.freshdesk.com and send us inquire, we will be glad to provide you an answer as quick as possible.

8.4 Dashboard

At the top of the screen you will find a navigation menu, it helps you access the different sections available in the solution (<u>*Dash*</u>), select or change locations, review, and erase notifications, adjust your account settings and log off. Note that *Users* do not have access to Administration Menu, only *Power Users* can access this feature (Fig. 8.5).

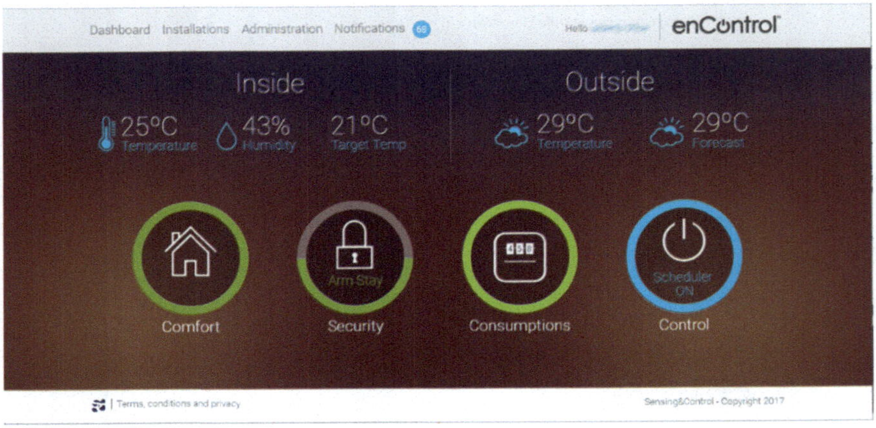

Fig. 8.5 Web application dashboard area

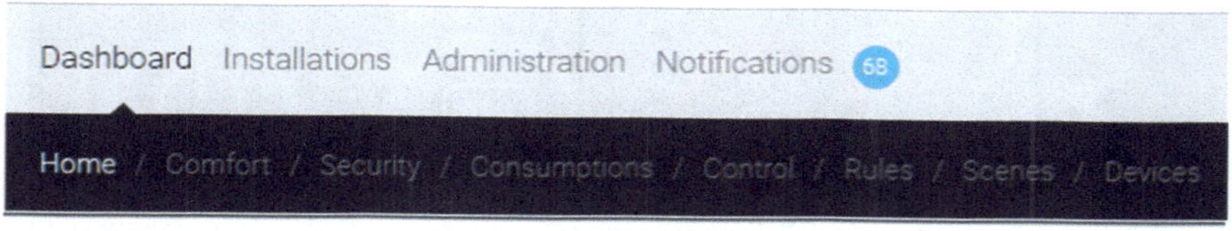

Fig. 8.6 Dashboard main subcategories

In the menu bar place your pointer over Dashboard, a sub-menu will appear. Move your pointer over the desired section (Comfort, Security, Consumptions, Control, Rules, Scenes and Devices) and click on it to access it. You can jump back and forward between sections anytime (Fig. 8.6).

A main Dashboard showing a status snapshot of your preferred default location will be presented to you. This screen provides a quick view of current conditions including climate, air quality, security, consumption performance and whether a routine for managing appliances or equipment has been scheduled (Fig. 8.7).

At the top left, you will find a quick view of comfort levels inside your selected location. *Temperature* indicates the current average measurements from all sensors installed. *Humidity* indicates the current average percentage of relative humidity in the air measured from all sensors within an area. *Target Temp*., indicates the temperature set point on your virtual thermostat—*ON* means that your heating or cooling system is working to reach and maintain the desired temperature; *OFF* means that your heating or cooling system has been turned off.

At the top right, you will see a quick view of current outside temperature and weather conditions in your area. This information comes from local weather sources and may not reflect the exact temperature in your neighborhood. You can also see the forecast temperature and weather conditions for your area.

An intuitive pallet of colors and simple messages updates you instantly about the current status of your installation. Messages and colors are displayed in later sections of this manual (Fig. 8.8).

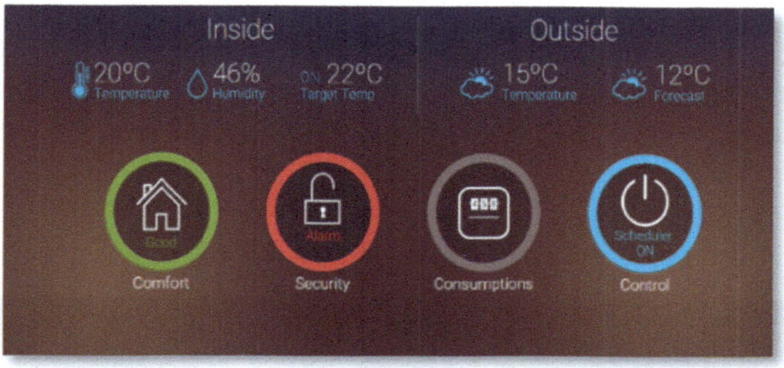

Fig. 8.7 Dashboard main information

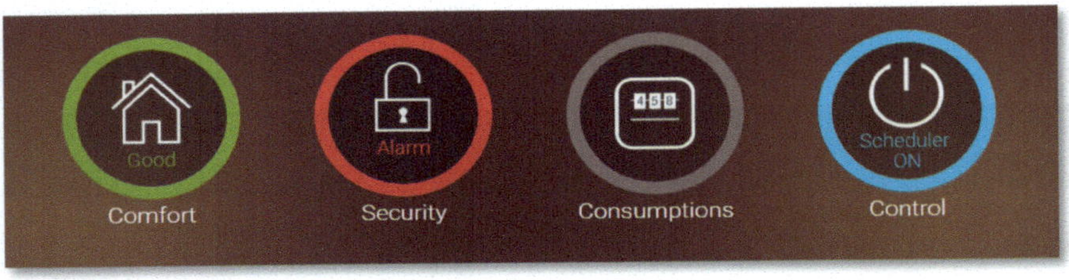

Fig. 8.8 Use of colors and simple messages at dashboard level

8.4.1 Notifications

To access detailed information on all incidents and events go to the *Dashboard* and click on the *Notifications* menu. A menu shows the number of unread notifications for each area. Click to get detailed information of events.

The notification events are divided in following concepts:

- **Security**—notifications related with security (like arm/disarm or alarms)
- **Comfort**—notifications related with comfort (like changing climate mode)
- **Consumption**—notifications related with energy consumption
- **Control** notifications related with control (like switching on/off a plug or light)
- **Devices**—notifications related with Device behavior (like offline/online)
- **System**—notifications related with system activities (like gateway restart or backup)
- **Custom**—personalized notifications by user (typically issued in rules/scenes) (Fig. 8.9).

8.4.2 Control Function

A set of different colors on the *Control* Icon will inform you of the current status of the automation functionalities. When the *General Scheduler* is turned *ON*, the *Control* icon on your *Dashboard* will display (Fig. 8.10).

Scheduler ON with blue coloring. You can manually turn *ON/OFF* or set automatic schedules for your equipment by clicking on the Icon.

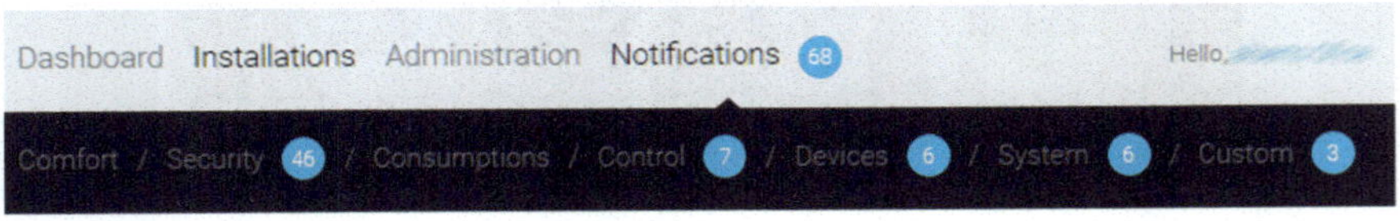

Fig. 8.9 Notifications main subcategories

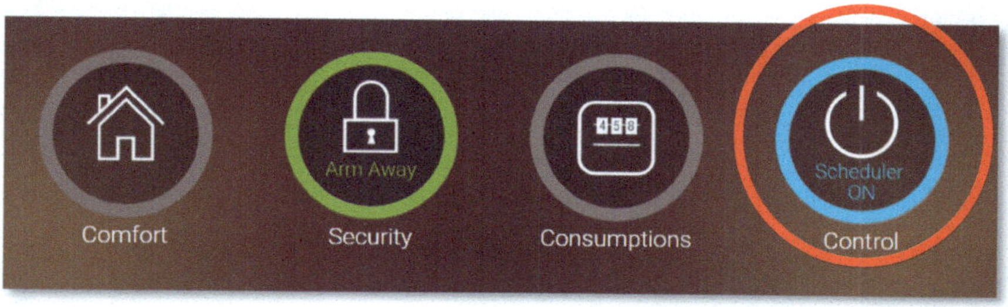

Fig. 8.10 Web application control functionality

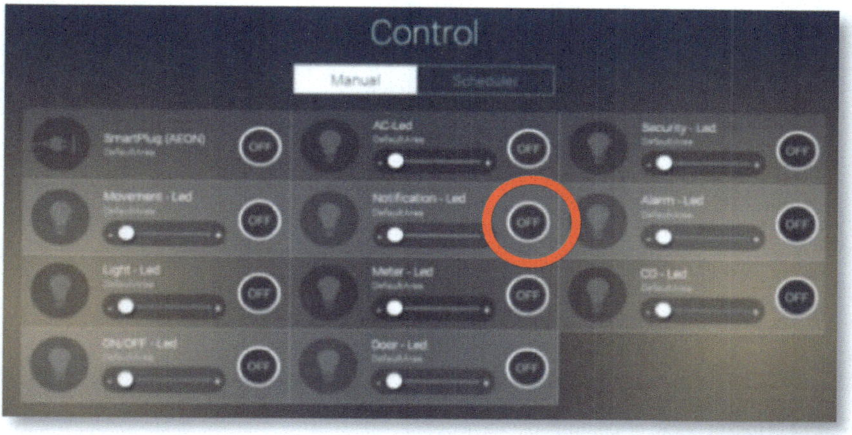

Fig. 8.11 Turning devices on/off

To turn *ON* or *OFF* equipment, appliances, lights, etc., just move your pointer over the selected device and click the *ON/OFF* circle (Fig. 8.11).

8.4.3 Devices Global View

The device view (sensors) gives you the global information of all of them in one shot. For each one you will be able to (Fig. 8.12):

1. Filter so that the view only shows the information that interests you, for example, by putting the name of an area, the view will only show the sensors assigned to that area.
2. See whether or not they are communicating with the gateway (the non-communicating device is labeled "Offline").

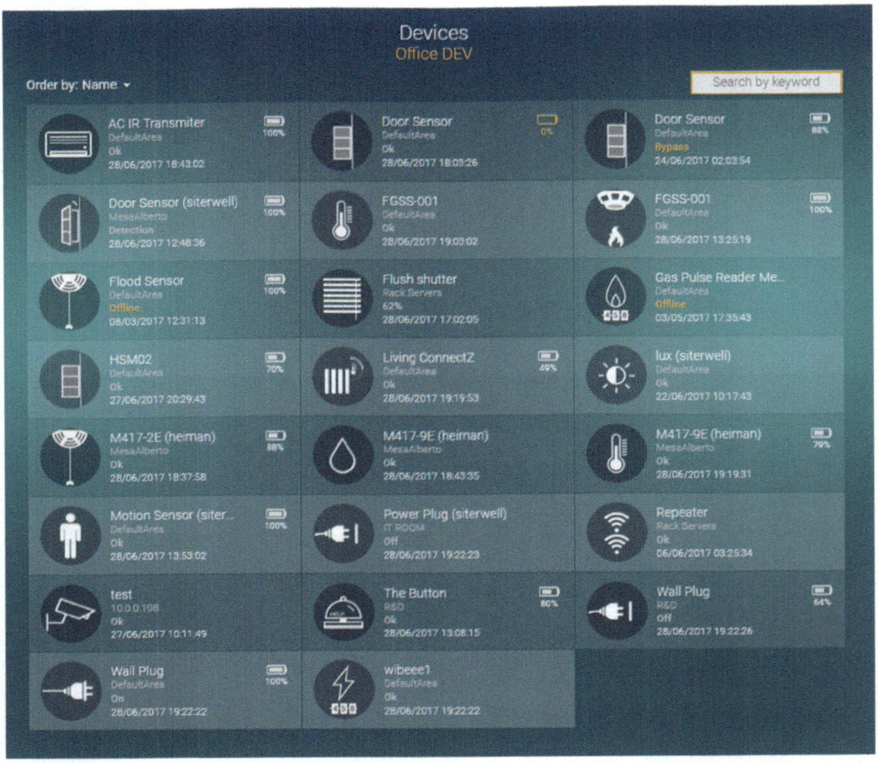

Fig. 8.12 Holistic view of controllable devices

3. You can know the date of last communication between the gateway and the sensor.
4. You can see the battery status reported by the device.
5. Clicking on a sensor you can display data and historical states through the dedicated view.

8.4.4 Rules

Once you have selected the "Rules" menu option you will be presented with a screen, where you can see the rules you already defined, and you can create new ones or disable, delete and modify the existing ones (see Fig. 8.13).

Once you have pressed " + add new rule," the following screen will appear, where you can

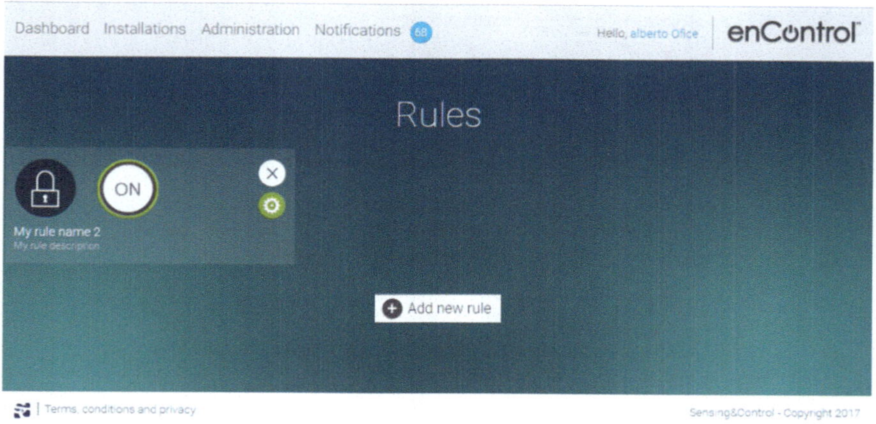

Fig. 8.13 Web application rule definition capabilities

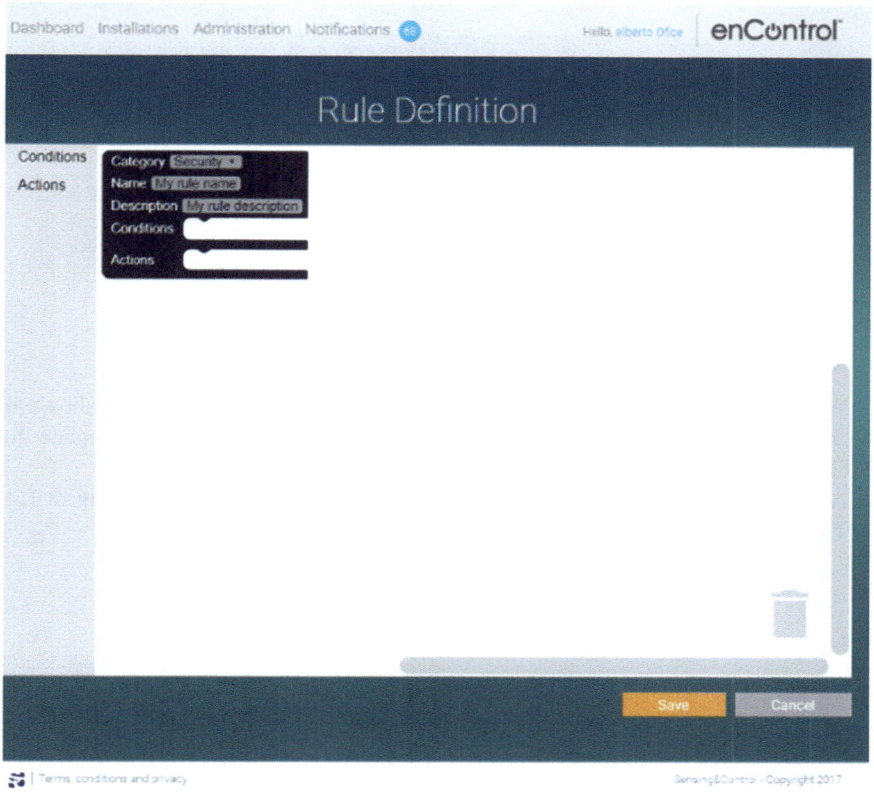

Fig. 8.14 Web application rule definition low complexity approach

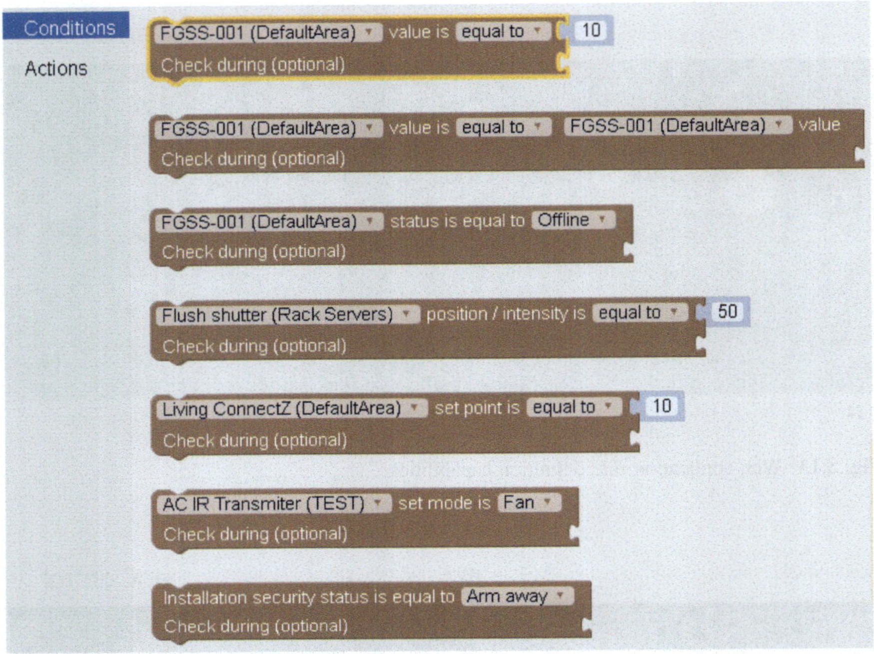

Fig. 8.15 Example of a rule's conditions

1. Select category (security, comfort, control, etc.)
2. Name it
3. Write a description
4. Select conditions
5. Select actions (Fig. 8.14).

When you select conditions, a series of preset selectors will appear, as shown in the following screenshot. You will have to select an option and stack it inside the "Conditions" slot.

All conditions must be met for the actions of the rule to be executed (Fig. 8.15).

The actions, like the conditions, are pre-configured (Fig. 8.16).

8.4.5 Scenes

Once you have selected the menu option "Scenes" you will be presented with a screen, where you can see the actions already defined, and you can create new ones or deactivate, delete and modify the existing ones (Fig. 8.17).

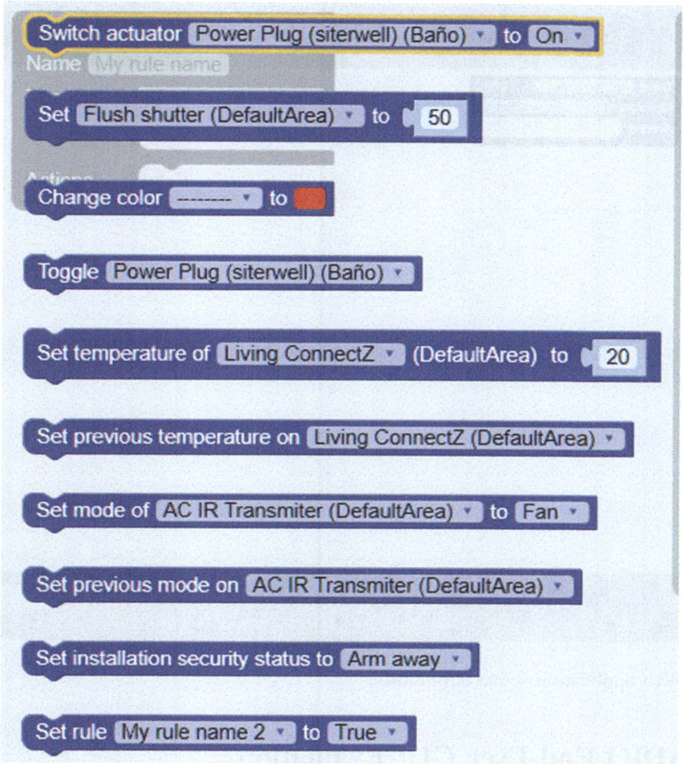

Fig. 8.16 Example of a rule's actions

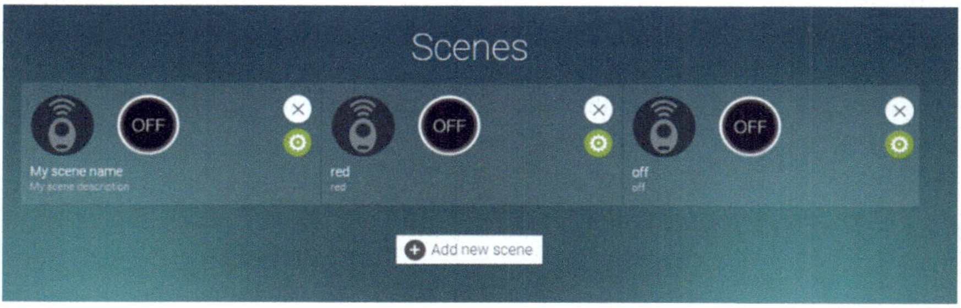

Fig. 8.17 Web application scene example

The execution of the scene is started by pressing the OFF button, at which time the execution request is made.

Once you click on " + add new scene," the following screen will appear, where you can give a name for the rule, give a description, and select the actions to be executed (as described in Rules section) (Fig. 8.18).

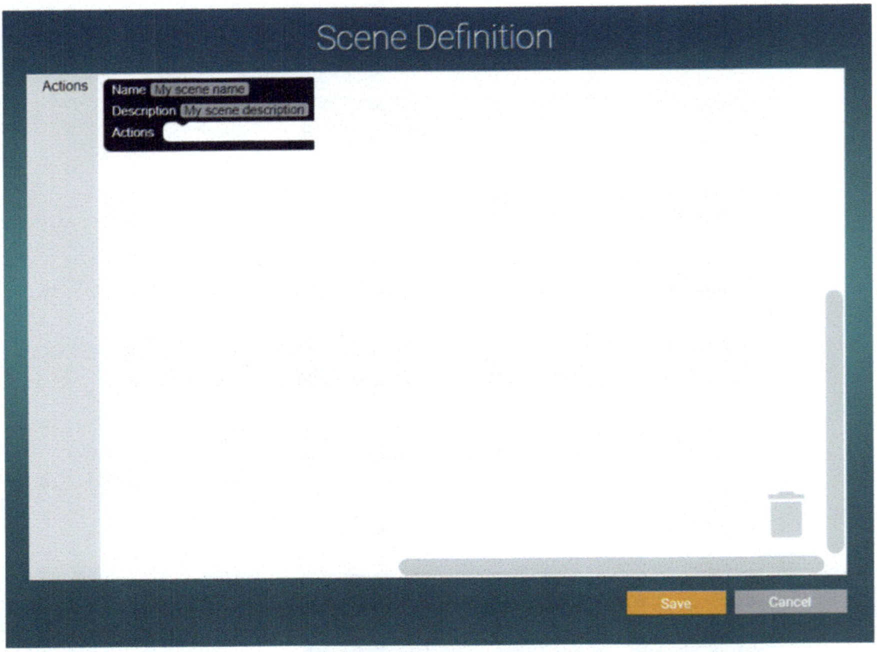

Fig. 8.18 Web application scene definition

8.5 RADIO End-User GUI Evaluation

This section describes the RADIO end-user GUI for controlling the robot via a multi-touch device (Android tablet or smartphone). The GUI is part of the RADIO end-user Android application. The main focus of this section is the evaluation methodology that has been applied comprising an expert evaluation and user testing using eye-tracking, as well as the conclusions reached.

8.5.1 RADIO End-User GUI

The main functionalities supported are: access to the Smart Home dashboard already discussed in Sect. 8.3, access to Facebook, robot control options and call for help. The scope of the evaluation comprises robot control options and call for help. The screenshots that follow were taken from an Android smartphone (Figs. 8.19, 8.20, 8.21, 8.22, 8.23 and 8.24).

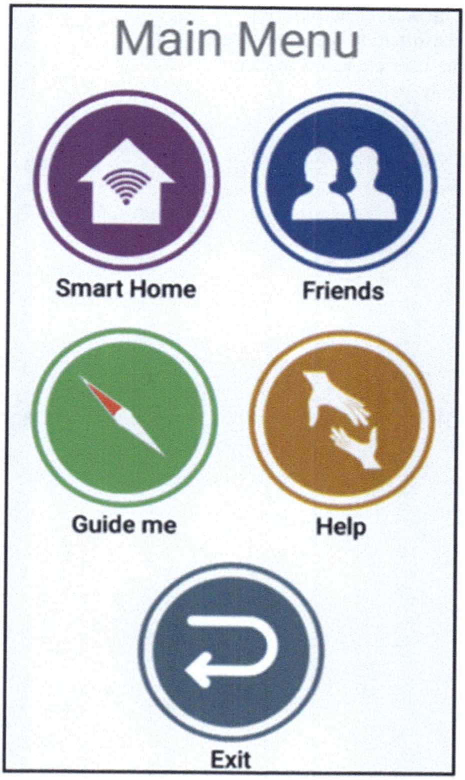

Fig. 8.19 The RADIO Main Menu screen

8.5.2 RADIO End-User GUI Evaluation

8.5.2.1 Expert Evaluation

The two expert evaluators examined the RADIO End-User GUI against the set of software guidelines for elderly users using multi-touch devices in Table 8.1 [18]. Evaluation assigns a symbol to each guideline depending on whether it is fully satisfied, partially satisfied or not satisfied by the RADIO End-User GUI:

● YES (the guideline is well-applied)

● YES but not fully (the guideline is applied to a degree, could be improved)

○ NO (the guideline is violated, improvements are required).

From the above it is concluded that the RADIO End-User GUI conforms to a high degree to the list of identified multi-touch UI guidelines for elderly users. More specifically, excluding 21 of the 58 guidelines that were considered non-applicable to the context of the RADIO application (see respective rationale on the preceding table), 35 from the remaining 37 guidelines are well-applied and 2 are applied but there is merit for further improvement.

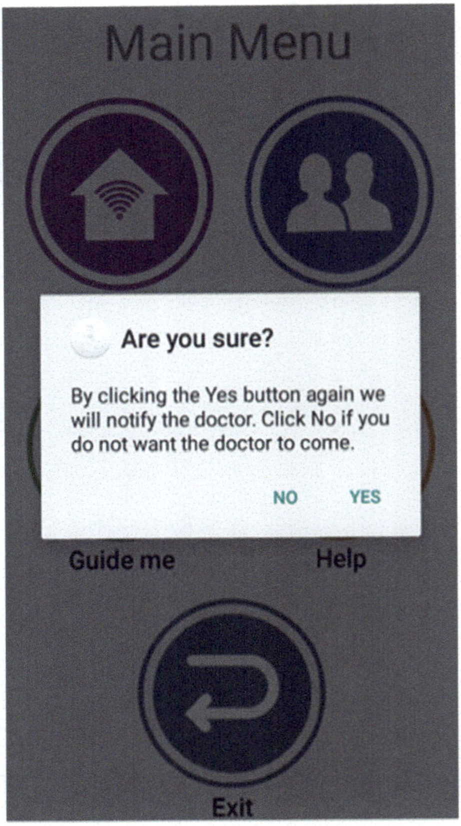

Fig. 8.20 The RADIO confirmation message when the user clicks on the Help icon

Summarizing the RADIO GUI conformance with the usability guidelines checklist, the GUI does not demonstrate any major or minor usability issues, but could be further enhanced if multiple line spacing is increased to 1.5 in text messages and if text sizes in general could be customizable to fit each user's needs (i.e. there is the option to adjust text sizes accordingly).

Another suggestion made by the evaluators is to unlock screen orientation so that the RADIO application can be used in landscape mode, too in the case of tablet devices. For smartphone usage, evaluators suggest to keep the screen locked to portrait orientation for better GUI layout.

Moreover, evaluators suggested increasing the spacing between screen contents and screen borders, as headings are placed too close to the top border of the screen and the labels of the "Back to Main Manu" and "Exit" buttons are too close to the bottom border of the screen.

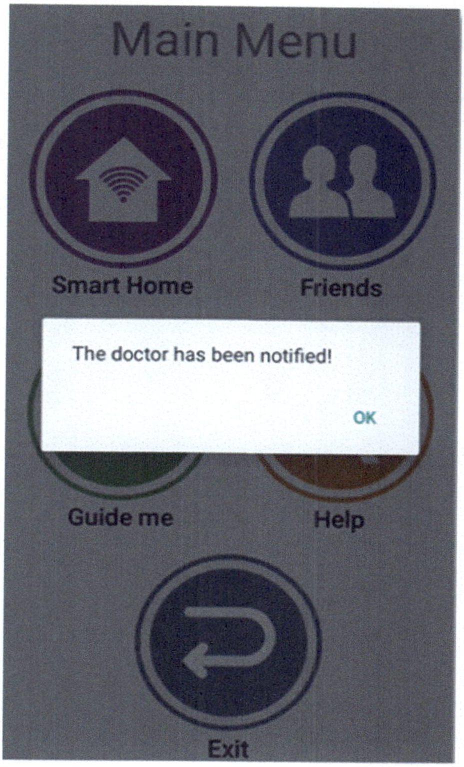

Fig. 8.21 The RADIO notification message when the user clicks YES on the confirmation message (Help icon clicked)

8.5.2.2 Eye-Tracking User Testing

Equipment

Eye tracking is a methodology that helps researchers understand visual attention. With eye tracking, we can detect where users look at a point in time, how long they look at something, and the path their eyes follow. It helps researchers understand the complete user experience, even that which users cannot describe [27]. Most modern eye-trackers rely on a method called corneal reflection to detect and track the location of the eye as it moves. Corneal reflection uses a light source to illuminate the eye, which then causes a reflection that is detected by a high-resolution camera. The image captured by the camera is then used to identify the reflection of the light source on the cornea and in the pupil. Advanced image processing algorithms are then used to establish the point of gaze related to the eye and the stimuli.

This process is divided into fixation and saccades. A fixation is the pause of the eye movement on a specific area of the visual field. Saccades are rapid movements of the eye from one fixation to another to help the eye piece together a complete

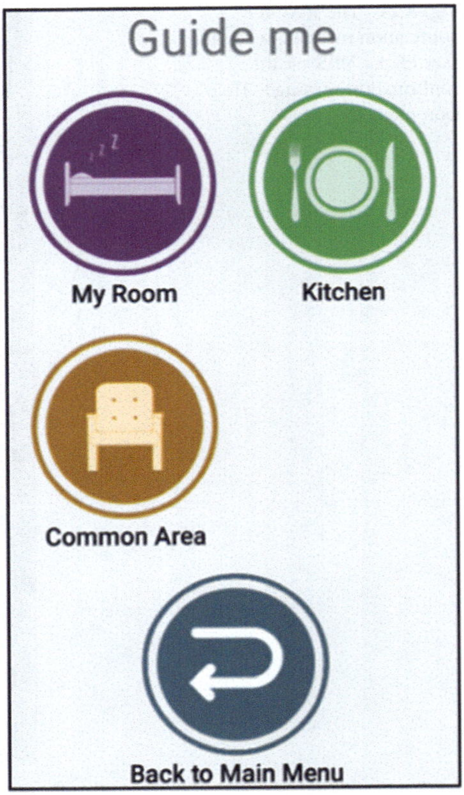

Fig. 8.22 The RADIO guide me screen (opens when the user clicks the 'Guide me' icon on the Main Menu screen)

scene of what an individual looks at. The eye-trackers that UX professionals use today come with software suites that instantaneously produce visualizations of the eye-tracking data and automate a significant amount of tasks that previously took weeks to analyze manually. The output from these software packages help to highlight where the user looked, the length of time they looked there, and the gaze pattern their eyes followed. Some of the most commonly used visualizations include the heat map and the gaze plot.

- A heatmap is a visualization that uses different colors to show the amount of fixations participants made or for how long they fixated on specific areas. Heat maps are color coded with areas with no color signifying that users may not have fixated on it. This does not necessarily mean they did not see anything—they may have looked there for a short period or may have only registered peripherally, but this is not detectable by the eye-tracker.
- Gaze plots are a visual representation of fixations and saccades for a particular time frame. In most software applications, fixations are represented by numbered dots, and saccades are lines connecting the dots. Fixations can vary in size to illustrate the duration of the fixation.

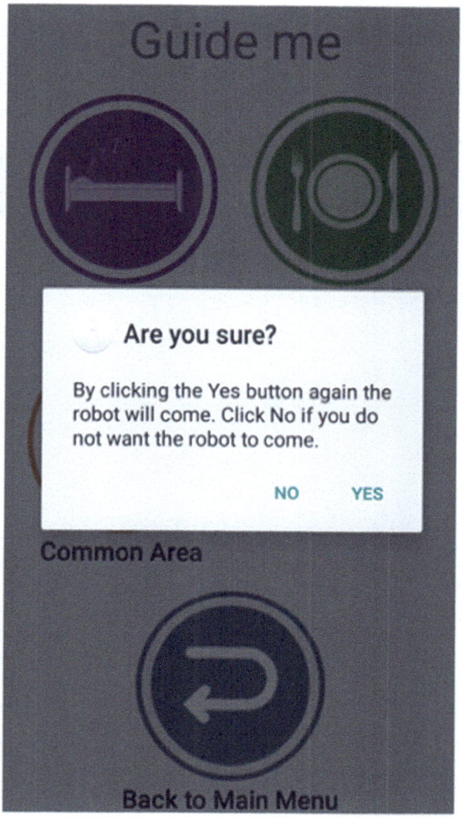

Fig. 8.23 The RADIO confirmation message when the user clicks on any of the 3 available icons (Bedroom, Kitchen or Common Area)

In the current study, eye-tracking has been used as a supportive means for validating icon recognizability and text readability as users are asked to performed specific tasks using the RADIO End-User GUI. The equipment used comprised

- **Tobii Glasses**: allow capturing free eye movement and fixation not just on a specific screen but anywhere in the environment surrounding the user. Data gathered by the eye-tracking glasses are much richer and can provide insights on what distracts users, for how long and how fast.
- **Tobii T60 Eye-Tracker**: integrated in a 17-in. TFT monitor, the eye-tracking system allows for a large degree of head movement, providing a distraction-free test environment that ensures natural behavior, and therefore valid results. The eye-tracking technology's high level of accuracy and precision ensures that the research results are reliable.
- **Tobii X60/X120 Mobile Device Testing Solution**: Allows eye tracking during natural interaction with smart phones, tablet computers or other devices or objects of similar size (up to 5 or 10 inches display). The device depending on

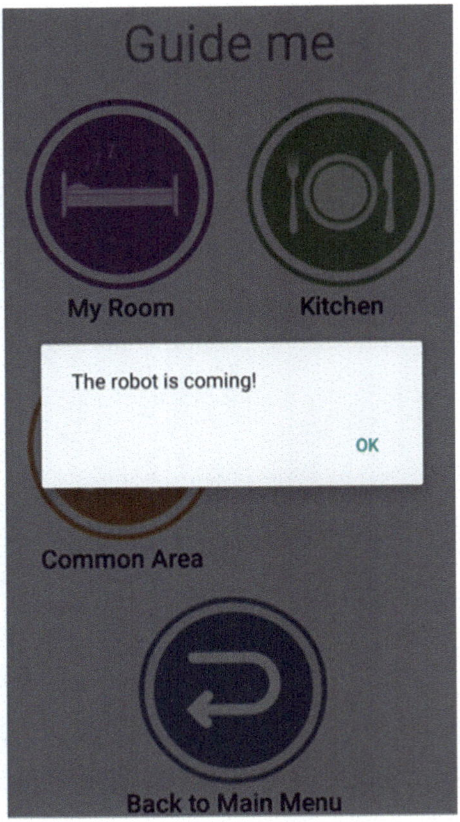

Fig. 8.24 The RADIO notification message when the user clicks YES on the confirmation message (Bedroom, Kitchen or Common Area icon clicked)

its size can be mounted either on the provided small device mount or on the large device mount. These mounts allow for smooth rotation of devices between landscape and portrait modes. The setup also allows for free hand movement testing where the device is not mounted but instead the participant holds it in his hands and leans against the setup's relevant surface (Figs. 8.25 and 8.26).

Collected data were processed by the Tobii studio software, a platform for stimuli presentation, recording, observation, visualization, and analysis of eye-tracking data. The software allows processing of large amounts of information for meaningful interpretation. More specifically, Tobii studio allows for designing eye-tracking usability studies, running test sessions, observing subjects remotely, visualizing the results, and analyzing statistics. It integrates a variety of data, besides eye tracking, to include stimuli presentation and subject behavior, which gives researchers a complete view of behavior. The software automatically synchronizes all of the data into one file (Fig. 8.27).

Replay of eye-tracking videos with the gaze point of the subject overlaid enables in-depth qualitative analysis and sharing of highlights. Tobii studio also generates

Table 8.1 Design guidelines for multi-touch interfaces for elderly users

	Guideline	Evaluation	Remarks
1	*DESIGN: color*		
1.1	Use colors of the long wavelength end of the spectrum (i.e., warm colors like red or yellow) if the color carries information—avoid blue especially	●	Color is used on icons (one color per each icon) for distinguishing reasons and when it is used on text it is confined to a shade of green. Blue is avoided as an information carrying color and it is only used on the Friends icon which corresponds to the Facebook brand color identity (as a hint to the application this icon opens)
1.2	Colors should be used conservatively. Use colors to carry important and relevant information (e.g., warnings, grouping elements)	●	Colors have been used in icons to provide distinguishability and in a monochrome fashion to avoid color pollution and overload
1.3	Keep in mind that dark background colors increase glare and highlight fingerprints	●	Background in native application screens is white
1.4	Avoid colored and patterned backgrounds for text display areas	●	All text display areas have a white background
DESIGN: contrast			
1.5	To ensure legibility the color contrast ratio of text smaller than 18 pt should be at least 7:1 or 4,5:1 for large text or decorative text	●	Color contrast ratio for text in button labels is 20.47:1 and for text on screen titles (larger text) is 6.62:1
DESIGN: typeface			
1.6	Use sans-serif font types (e.g., Verdana or Arial)	●	All texts in the application are in a sans-serif font
1.7	Avoid decorative, italic, underlined and condensed font styles. Use bold font types and uppercase text only for highlighting key terms	●	Bold, italic, or otherwise decorated font formatting has been avoided throughout the application
2	*LAYOUT: size and spacing*		
2.1	Buttons, clickable icons and labels should range in size between 11.43 mm square minimum and 19.05 mm square maximum. Adjacent buttons used in rows (e.g., keypad) should be at least 16.51 mm square	●	Both metric ranges are respected in all buttons, icons and labels

(continued)

Table 8.1 (continued)

	Guideline	Evaluation	Remarks
2.2	The spacing between adjacent buttons in a row should reach from 3.17 to 12.7 mm maximum	●	Icon spacing conforms to the guideline
2.3	Font sizes for multiple line text (i.e., primary text) should range between 9 and 14 pt and depend on screen size and the visual acuity of the user	●	Multiline text is used only in informative messages and messages for action verification. Text size in these messages is between 9 and 14 pt
2.4	A 1.5 line spacing up to double spacing increases readability of text	● (grey)	Text in informative text messages (the only case where text wraps in many lines) is readable but a 1.5 line spacing could improve its readability even more
LAYOUT: text layout			
2.5	Keep text lines short in length: the amount of characters per line for primary text should range between 60 and 75	●	Text lines' length conforms to the guideline
2.6	Avoid the need of scrolling to read a text. Rather consider to decrease the font size or line spacing	●	No scrolling is required
2.7	Avoid moving text like automatic scrolling	●	No scrolling is required
2.8	Multiple line text should be left justified	●	Text alignment conforms to the guideline
2.9	Provide clear and large headings	●	All screens have a large and clear heading indicating the current position in the application
LAYOUT: content structure			
2.10	Simplicity of visual perception is key: avoid visual clutter, distracting visual stimuli and non-relevant information due to the declining visual field	●	Visual elements are kept to a minimum, there are no decorative elements, screens have enough white space (especially in the tablet version) and visual elements are used to represent clickable icons of the application
2.11	Minimize working memory demands: keep the number of information blocks presented or processed at once limited to around 5	●	In all native application screens available options are kept to a maximum of 5

(continued)

Table 8.1 (continued)

	Guideline	Evaluation	Remarks
LAYOUT: consistency			
2.12	Consistent design is even more important for the elderly than it is for younger people. Therefore, the location of items and functions should remain the same across views and similar functions should act the same way throughout the application	●	Consistency is respected and kept in all screens (same buttons have the same behavior, representation and positioning, text in message screens keep consistent phrasing and options)
LAYOUT: navigation and menu structure			
2.13	Group information and actions into meaningful and clearly worded categories. The difference between the options should be apparent	●	Options are coded into different colors and icons are large and contain a distinguishing graphic. Grouping is not applicable as options are limited to 5 (maximum)
2.14	Provide a clear and consistent navigation by displaying precise navigation cues and actions that are readily visible and accessible	●	Each screen has a clear title and an option for returning to the previous one
2.15	The current location in the application should be obvious to the user all the time	●	Each screen has a clear title
2.16	Avoid deep hierarchies in menu structures hence the user does not get lost in the application	●	The application has a very simple and shallow structure, which ensures that in no point the user might feel disoriented or lost
2.17	Minimize the number of steps to complete a task as well as the number of control-elements to increase the probability of successfully completing the task	●	All tasks can be accomplished in a sequence of 3 clicks (provided that the user makes no mistakes)
2.18	Don't force the user to keep information in mind for too long to accomplish a single task	●	The user does not need to remember any information to accomplish a task (just to have in mind the task itself)
3	*Language and wording*		
3.1	Language should be simple and clear. In addition, it should use active voicing and positive phrasing	●	Language is simple without any technical references. It uses active voicing and positive phrasing

(continued)

Table 8.1 (continued)

	Guideline	Evaluation	Remarks
3.2	Phrasing assuming prior knowledge (e.g., technical terms) or a certain (especially young) age of the user should be avoided. Provide a glossary if technical terms are necessary	●	Language is simple without any technical references. No need to provide a glossary
4	*Icons, graphics and multimedia*		
4.1	Well designed or familiar symbols and icons can be more effective ways to convey information than text messages	●	Icons have a representative and distinguishing graphic seniors are familiar with
4.2	Where possible provide a label or text for icons or illustrated instructions	●	All icons are accompanied by a textual label
4.3	Speech rate of verbal information should be kept to 140 words per minute or less, male voices should be preferred to female voices and synthesized speech should be as natural as possible	Non-applicable	The application does not support speech
4.4	Consider providing parallel visual and auditory presentation of language (i.e., subtitles or a text-to-speech function)	Non-applicable	The application does not support speech
4.5	Limit your sounds to one at a time; for example, speech over music may be hard to distinguish	●	Sounds are restricted to system sounds that act as feedback when an action needs confirmation
5	*INTERACTION: gestures and data entry*[a]	Non-applicable	
INTERACTION: feedback			
5.15	Support the user by indicating the touch location with visual feedback	●	Touch locations are clearly indicated by large sized icons the users can simply click (tap) to activate
5.16	Use low frequency vibration (25–60 Hz) for vibrotactile feedback	Non-applicable	No vibration is used as a feedback mechanism
5.17	Auditory feedback should provide a volume of at least 60 dB and a sound-frequency of 500–2000 Hz. If high frequencies have to be used the duration (at least 500 ms) should be increased	●	Auditory feedback conforms to the guideline
5.18	Multi-modal (combining audio, visual and/or tactile signals) feedback should be favored over unimodal feedback. Especially tactile and visual feedback should not be used solely	●	All visual feedback is used in combination with audio feedback

(continued)

Table 8.1 (continued)

	Guideline	Evaluation	Remarks
5.19	Provide ample time to process information and to make a physical response	●	There is no time limit for users to proceed with any action within the application
5.20	Provide error messages that are informative about the error occurred, the consequences and how to recover from it. Error messages should always appear at the same location	●	Error messages appear the same way informative or verification messages appear (see section 5), i.e. in a white panel in the center of the screen while graying-out the preceding screen
6	USER support and training	Non-applicable	
7	*Personalization*		
7.1	Adjusting certain factors of an user interface (e.g., the font size) to personal needs is important for the elderly	● (grey)	Font sizes are large enough. Nevertheless it would be good to allow for adjusting font sizes
7.2	Consider to make some of the following factors adjustable: the size of font, graphics or targets the combination of audio, tactile and visual feedback the way data is entered (software or physical keyboard) the range of application functionalities style information like background images or colors	●	See 7.1 comment Visual and audio feedback are already combined There is no need for data entry in all native application screens There is no additional functionality to be gradually introduced Style could be adjusted but allowing only predefined combinations to ensure contrast guidelines are met. In this case though it is doubtful if the option for customizing the style justifies the extra effort seniors will have to put in order to manipulate an additional GUI feature

[a]The native application screens require no data entry (the application is connected to a dashboard app and Facebook but the evaluation of those UIs is not part of this study)

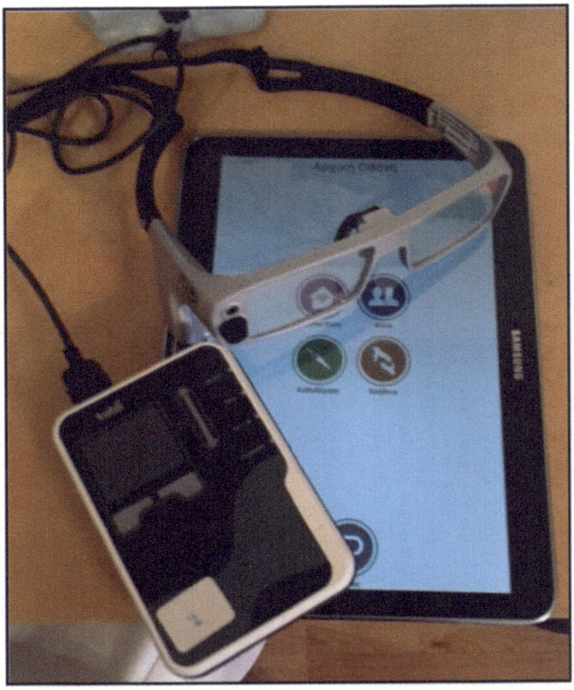

Fig. 8.25 Tobii eye-tracking glasses used for RADIO UI evaluation

overview of the data for a more detailed quantitative analysis and interpretation by using the calculation of eye tracking and click metrics based on AOI's (Areas Of Interest), as well as versatile tables and charts. Raw or filtered eye-tracking data can be exported for further analysis and significance testing in Excel, SPSS, MATLAB, and other statistical software suites. In addition, adjustable fixation filters are available for eye movement classifications.

User testing sessions were video recorded using a SONY HXR-NX30E wide 10 × optical video camera and photographs were taken using a Canon EOS50D camera with an extra zoom lens EF24-70MM 1:2,8.

Methodology

For the purposes of user testing a series of 10 home visits were scheduled. In every visit two usability experts were present moderating the tests and specialized personnel from Frontida Zois were overlooking the process. The test was performed at the premises of the elderly at a prearranged date and time according to the preferences of each user.

Users were initially informed about the RADIO project aims and expected results and were informed about the experiment process and the estimated duration. Then, each user was asked to sign off a consensus form for video recording and photos and to provide information regarding age and previous experience with tablets/smartphones/PCs. Regarding user demographics, the majority of users were

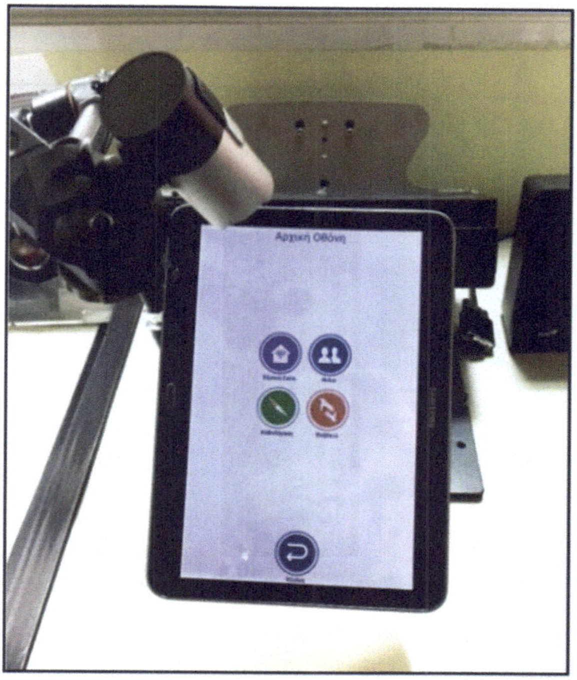

Fig. 8.26 Tobii eye-tracker mounted on a mobile device stand

female (80%) and 30% of them were less than 65 years old, 30% were 66–70 years old and 40% were from 71 to 80 years old. When asked about their previous usage experience with tablets/smartphones/PCs 20% of users responded that they have experience with all three devices (half of them also use Facebook), 30% stated that they have only used tablets and 30% that they have no relative prior experience. After this initial stage of the session users were shown the Main Menu screen (Fig. 8.19) and then the Guide Me screen (Fig. 8.22) in order to get familiar with their contents and layout and then to perform the scenarios in Table 8.2.

After collecting all data previously described, they were analyzed to provide descriptive statistics regarding the test and qualitative information about the RADIO application evaluation.

Collected data and analysis

As previously mentioned, users were asked to observe the two main screens (Main Menu and Guide Me) without having yet specified any tasks.

The Heatmap revealed that the first line icons (purple and blue) were noticed more by users which can be justified by their position and color. Western world reading pattern (from left to right and from top to bottom) explains the sequence of eye-fixations on the gaze plot. Both representations indicate that all centrally located icons gathered the visual attention of users (Fig. 8.28).

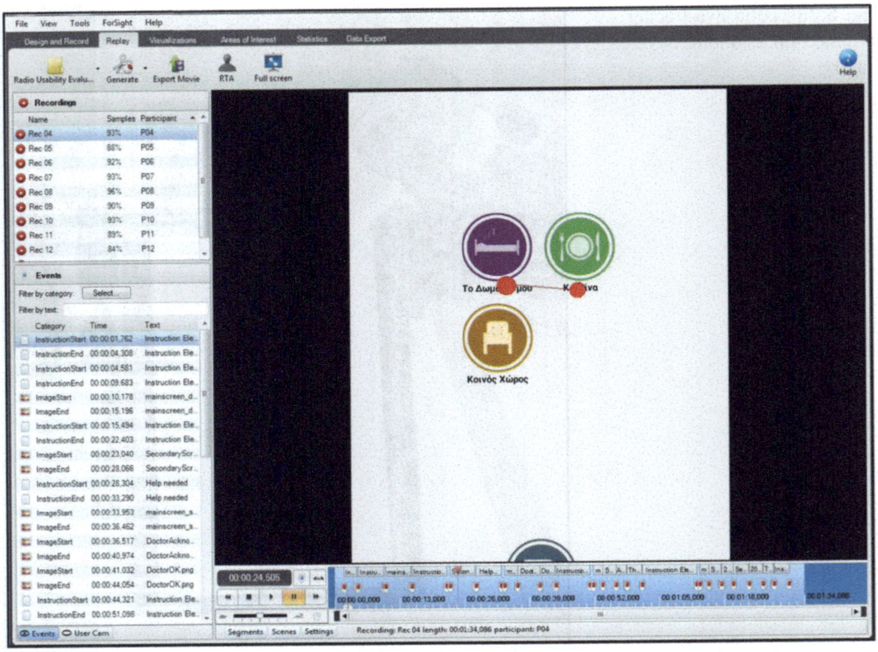

Fig. 8.27 Tobii Studio screenshot from the RADIO UI evaluation

Table 8.2 User test scenarios

	Scenarios	Evaluation objectives
1	[The user is at the Main Menu screen]: click the appropriate icon to call the doctor and confirm your action when asked to	'Help' icon recognizability Readability and understandability of confirmation text message Size suitability of confirmation message options ('No', 'Yes', 'OK')
2	[The user is at the Main Menu screen]: call the robot to guide you to the Kitchen and confirm your action when asked to	'Guide me' icon recognizability 'Kitchen' icon recognizability Size suitability of confirmation message options ('No', 'Yes', 'OK')
3	[The user is at the Main Menu screen]: call the robot to guide you to the Common Area, cancel your selection when asked to confirm it and then ask the robot to guide you to the bedroom (and confirm when asked to)	'Guide me' icon memorability 'Common Area' icon recognizability Readability and understandability of confirmation text message Readability and understandability of cancelation text message 'My Room' icon recognizability Size suitability of confirmation message options ('No', 'Yes', 'OK')

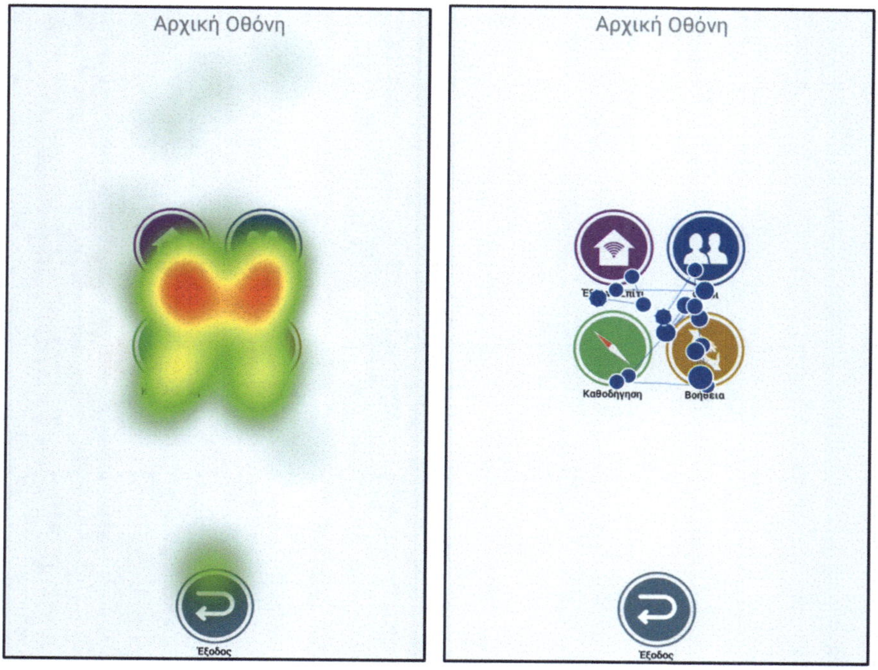

Fig. 8.28 Main Menu screen Heatmap (gaze data from all users) and Gaze plot (indicatively, one user)

The same observations hold in the case of users observing the Guide Me (Fig. 8.22) screen. The icon on the left topmost position is more noticed by users but they also gaze on the other two icons. Again users seem not to notice the headings, which is rather an indication that icons have a predominant role and that users will only look for headings in case they lose their direction (this is something to be examined during the scenarios).

In scenario 1, users were asked to (a) click the appropriate icon to call the doctor and (b) confirm their action when asked to (Fig. 8.29).

Users have recognized the correct icon after observing all icons, no user clicked on a "wrong" icon and users also reacted as expected when they were shown the confirmation message (read the text and the options and selected the one indicated by the scenario). Thus eye-tracking data have confirmed "Help" icon recognizability, readability and understandability of confirmation text message, and size suitability of confirmation messages options ("No," "Yes," and "OK").

In scenario 2, users were asked to (a) call the robot, (b) ask to guide them to the Kitchen and (c) confirm the action when asked to.

Users have recognized the "Guide me" icon after observing a limited set of icons (Fig. 8.30). That means that at a very early stage of their interaction experience, they recognize and recall the correct icon. In the second screen the "Kitchen" icon

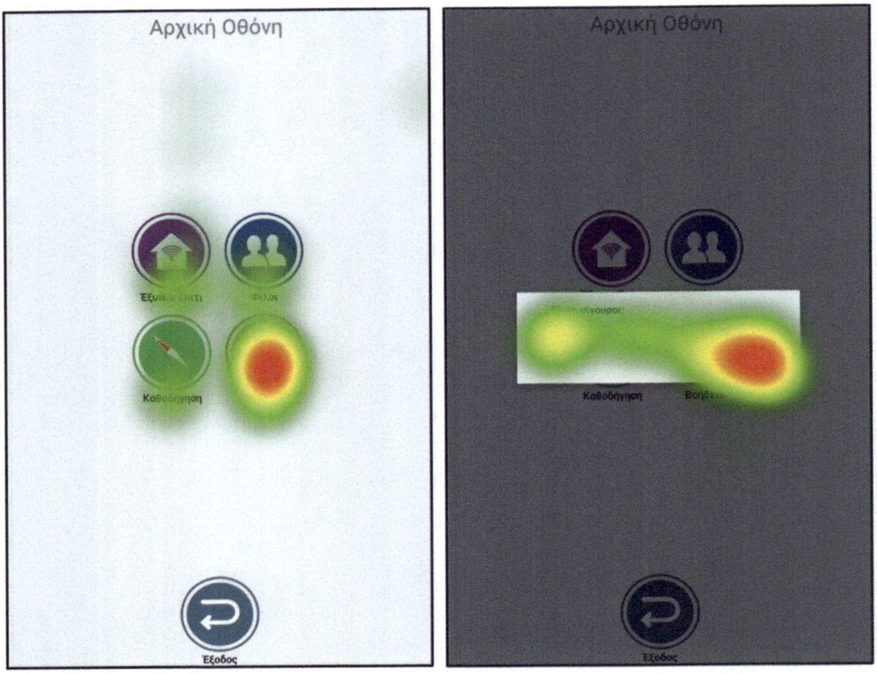

Fig. 8.29 Heatmap of step 1 (click on button to call the doctor) and step 2 (confirm that you want to call the doctor), gaze data from all users for scenario 1

was easily located and selected by all users. No user clicked on a "wrong" icon and users also reacted as expected when they were shown the confirmation message (read the text and the options and selected the one indicated by the scenario). Thus data collected by the eye-tracker have confirmed "Guide me" icon recognizability, "Kitchen" icon recognizability, and size suitability of confirmation messages options ("No," "Yes," and "OK").

In scenario 3, users were asked to (a) call the robot to guide them to the Common Area, (b) cancel their action when asked to confirm it, (c) ask the robot to guide them to the bedroom and (d) confirm when asked.

Eye-tracking data for step 1 resembled closely the visualization in Fig. 8.30. Seniors fixated longer on the Guide Me icon and that was their final selection (click). Next, users were should select the Common Area icon. Figure 8.31 confirms that users fixated and finally clicked on the requested icon.

Users seem to be very familiar with the main screen of RADIO. The "Guide me" icon was easily selected. Users have recognized the "Common Room" icon after a very limited number of fixations in other icons. That means that at a very early stage of their interaction experience, they recognize and recall the correct icon. Quite similar is the case with the "My Room" icon, although users seem to spend more time looking around (the number of fixations is bigger than the previous two cases).

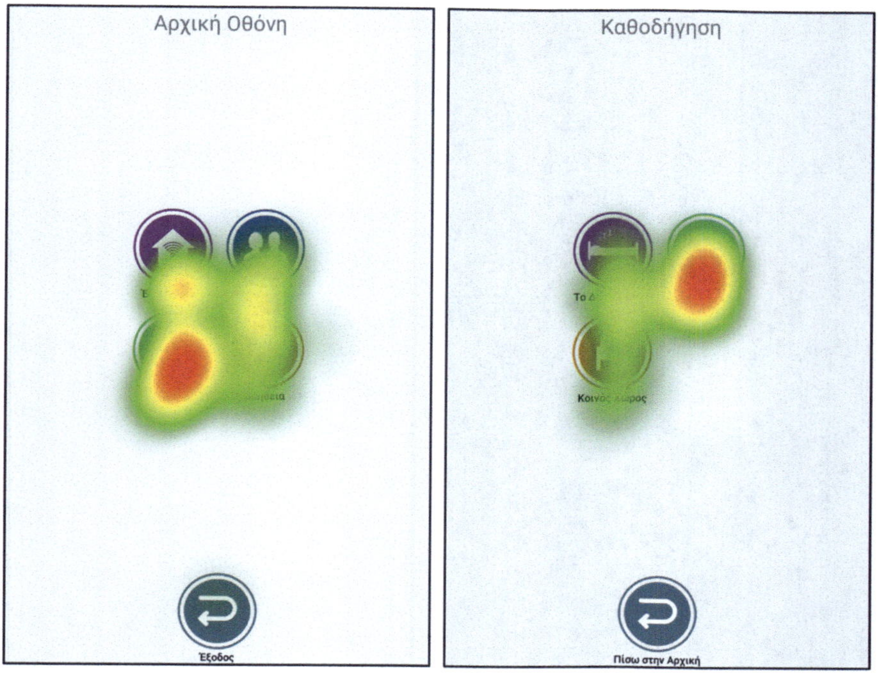

Fig. 8.30 Heatmap of step 1 (call the robot to guide you to the kitchen), and step 2 (select the kitchen), gaze data from all users for scenario 2

But no user clicked on a "wrong" icon and users also reacted as expected when they were shown the confirmation message (read the text and the options and selected the one indicated by the scenario).

8.6 Conclusion

The RADIO project addresses elderly users, a population that is growing steadily the last decades worldwide and especially in the developed countries. This part of the population faces limitations that typically include reduced visual ability, hearing loss, psychomotor impairments, loss of fine motor control, attention-related problems, and learning and memory impairments, characteristics that impose a number of additional challenges when trying to guarantee usability. This chapter presented the RADIO GUI emphasizing on the interaction and user interface guidelines that guided the design decisions and on the applied evaluation methodology and findings. The RADIO End-User GUI addresses seniors for allowing them to control the robot via a multi-touch device and is part of the RADIO end-user Android application. It was evaluated by two usability experts using heuristic evaluation and a set

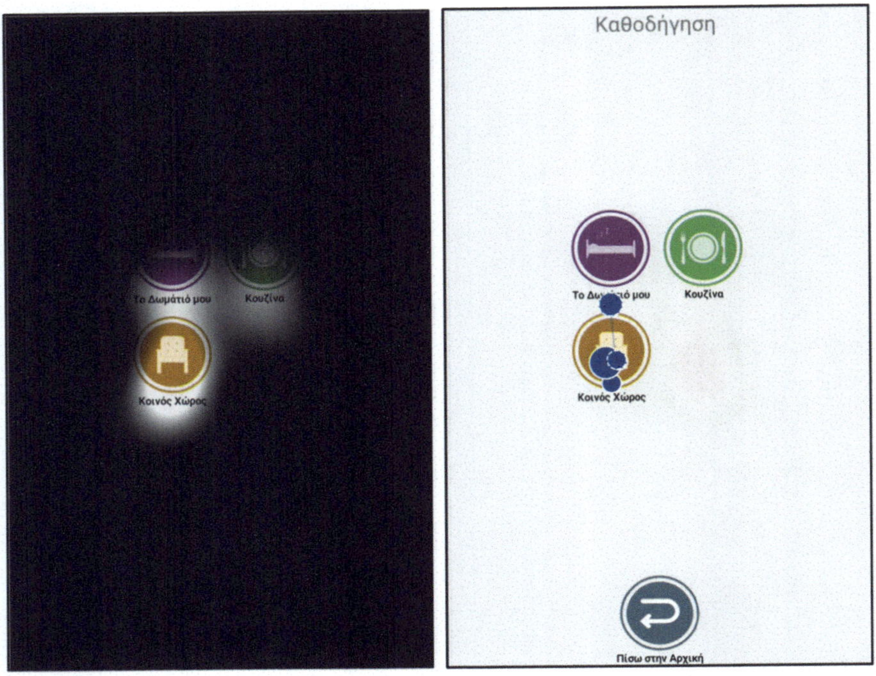

Fig. 8.31 Opacity heatmap (gaze data from all users) and Gaze plot (indicatively, one user) of step 2 (select the Common Area) for scenario 3

of guidelines for elderly users using applications on multi-touch devices. In addition, the system was evaluated by users executing specific scenarios that were eye-tracked. Expert evaluation concluded that the system conforms to a high degree to the list of guidelines (35 from the remaining 37 guidelines are well-applied and 2 are applied but there was a small merit for further improvement). User testing and mainly data collected by the eye-tracker have confirmed recognizability and memorability of icons as well as readability and understandability of textual content.

References

1. United Nations, Department of Economic and Social Affairs, & Population Division. (2017). World population ageing 2017—Highlights (ST/ESA/SER.A/397).
2. Zaphiris, P., Ghiawadwala, M., & Mughal, S. (2005). Age-centered research-based web design guidelines. In *CHI'05 Extended Abstracts on Human Factors in Computing Systems (Portland, OR, USA, April 02–07, 2005)* (pp. 1897–1900). New York, NY: ACM.
3. Stößel, C. (2012). *Gestural interfaces for elderly users: Help or hindrance?* Ph.D. thesis, Technische Universität Berlin, Berlin.

4. Hart, T. A., Chaparro, B. S., & Halcomb, C. G. (2008). Evaluating websites for older adults: Adherence to 'senior-friendly' guidelines and end-user performance. *Behaviour & Information Technology, 27*(3), 191–199. https://doi.org/10.1080/01449290600802031.
5. Hawthorn, D. (2000). Possible implications of aging for interface designers. *Interacting with Computers, 12*(5), 507–528. https://doi.org/10.1016/S0953-5438(99)00021-1.
6. Finn, K., & Johnson, J. (2013) A usability study of websites for older travelers. In: C. Stephanidis & M. Antona (Eds.), *Lecture notes in computer science: Vol. 8010. Universal access in human-computer interaction. User and context diversity. UAHCI 2013*. Berlin, Heidelberg: Springer.
7. World Wide Web Consortium (W3C). (n.d.). *Web content accessibility guidelines (WCAG) 2.1, W3C candidate recommendation 30 January 2018*. http://www.w3.org/TR/WCAG.
8. Carmien S., Manzanares, A. G. (2014). Elders using smartphones—A set of research based heuristic guidelines for designers. In *International conference on universal access in human-computer interaction* (pp. 26–37). Berlin: Springer.
9. Ijsselsteijn, W., Nap, H. H., de Kort, Y., & Poels, K. (2007). Digital game design for elderly users. In *Proceedings of the 2007 conference on future play* (pp. 17–22). ACM.
10. Nielsen, J. (1994). Heuristic evaluation. In J. Nielsen & R. L. Mack (Eds.), *Usability inspection methods*. New York, NY: Wiley.
11. Sibley, C. (2008). Web Usability and Aging. Article available from https://www.usability.gov/get-involved/blog/2008/12/aging-and-usability.htm.
12. Wood, E., Willoughby, T., Rushing, A., Bechtel, L., & Gilbert, J. (2005). Use of computer input devices by older adults. *Journal of Applied Gerontology, 24*(5), 419–438. https://doi.org/10.1177/0733464805278378.
13. Caprani, N., O'Connor, N. E., & Gurrin, C. (2012). Touch screens for the older user. In F. A. Cheein (Ed.), *Assistive technologies* (pp. 104–128). Ireland: Intech. March 2012. https://doi.org/10.5772/38302.
14. Lepicard, G., & Vigouroux, N. (2012). *Lecturers Notes Computer science: Computers Helping People with Special Needs, Vol. 7382, No. PART 1. Comparison between singletouch and multi-touch interaction for older people* (pp. 658–665). https://doi.org/10.1007/978-3-642-31522-0_99
15. Teiche, A., Rai, A. K., Yanc, C., Moore, C., Solms, D., Çetin, G., et al. (2009). *Multi-touch technologies* (p. 100). NUI Group.
16. Nielsen, J., & Molich, R. (1990). Heuristic evaluation of user interfaces. In *Proceedings of ACM CHI'90 Conference* (Seattle, WA, 1–5 April) (pp. 249–256).
17. Fisk, A. D., Rogers, W. A., Charness, N., Czaja, S. J., & Sharit, J. (2009). *Human factors & aging series. Designing for older adults: Principles and creative human factors approaches* (2nd ed). Boca Raton, FL: CRC Press. ISBN: 978-1-4200-8055 (Google Inc.).
18. Blendinger, K. (2015). *Tablet-applications for the elderly: Specific usability guidelines*. Master thesis, Faculty of Engineering and Computer Science, Ulm University, Germany.
19. Farage, M. A., Miller, K. W., Ajayi, F., & Hutchins, D. (2012). Design principles to accommodate older adults. *Global Journal of Health Science, 4*(2), 2–25. ISSN: 1916-9736. https://doi.org/10.5539/gjhs.v4n2p2.
20. Chadwick-Dias, A., McNulty, M., &Tullis, T. S. (2002). Web usability and age: How design changes can improve performance. *ACM SIGCAPH Computers and the Physically Handicapped* (Issue 73–74, pp 30–37). ISSN: 0163-5727. https://doi.org/10.1145/960201.957212. URL http://doi.acm.org/10.1145/960201.957212.
21. Tullis, T. S. (2007). Older adults and the web: Lessons learned from eye-tracking. In *Lecture notes in computer science: Vol. 4554. Universal acess in human computer interaction. Coping with diversity* (pp. 1030–1039). Berlin Heidelberg: Springer. ISBN: 978-3-540-73278-5. URL: https://doi.org/10.1007/978-3-540-73279-2_115.
22. Nielsen, J. (2013). Seniors as web users, 2013. URL: http://www.nngroup.com/.
23. Kobayashi, M., Hiyama, A., Miura, T., Asakawa, C., Hirose, M., & Ifukube, T. (2011). Elderly user evaluation of mobile touchscreen interactions. In *Lecture notes in computer science, human-computer interaction: Vol. 6946. INTERACT 2011* (pp 83–99). Berlin

Heidelberg: Springer. ISBN: 978-3-642- 23773-7. https://doi.org/10.1007/978-3-642-23774-4_9. URL http://dx.doi.org/10.1007/978-3-642-23774-4_9.
24. Loureiro, B., & Rodrigues, R. (2014). Design guidelines and design recommendations of multi-touch interfaces for elders. In *ACHI 2014, The Seventh International Conference on Advances in Computer-Human Interactions* (pp. 41–47).
25. Farage, L. G., Vigouroux, N., & Gorce, P. (2013). Interaction techniques for older adults using touchscreen devices: A literature review. In *Proceedings of the 25th IEME Conference Francophone on L'Interaction Homme-Machine, IHM'13* (pp. 125:125–125:134). New York, NY, USA: ACM. ISBN: 978-1-4503-2407-6. http://doi.acm.org/10.1145/2534903.2534920.
26. Campbell, O. (2015). *Designing for the elderly: Ways older people use digital technology differently, 2015*. Available online: https://www.smashingmagazine.com/2015/02/designing-digital-technology-for-the-elderly/.
27. Bergstrom J. R., & Schall, A. (2014). *Eye tracking in user experience design* (1st ed.). San Francisco, CA, USA: Morgan Kaufmann Publishers Inc.

Chapter 9
The Ecosystem of Connected RADIO Systems

Angelos Charalambidis, Giannis Mouchakis and Stasinos Konstantopoulos

9.1 Introduction

RADIO home deployments live and act inside the *RADIO ecosystem*. The RADIO home deployments integrate seamlessly in the RADIO ecosystem as nodes to an abstract network regardless of the different communication technologies and of the heterogeneous hardware and software components that comprise them.

The RADIO ecosystem provides the necessary mix of components and interconnections in order to support useful operations such as clinical report inspection, privacy-preserving data analysis, notifications, and home automation. These operations must comply with requirements regarding the protection of the sensitive data produced in each RADIO home.

This design aims to place the local network of each RADIO home in the overall context of the RADIO ecosystem of communicating RADIO homes, caregivers, and care institutions; and to do so in a way that

- Allows only relevant information to be shared and ensures the security of private data and extracted information;
- Can scale to a large number of RADIO home deployments managed by a single-care institution; and
- Can handle heterogeneity in communication technologies and hardware and software components.

A. Charalambidis (✉) · G. Mouchakis · S. Konstantopoulos
Institute of Informatics and Telecommunications, NCSR "Demokritos", Aghia Paraskevi, Greece
e-mail: acharal@iit.demokritos.gr

V. Karkaletsis et al. (eds.), *RADIO–Robots in Assisted Living*,
https://doi.org/10.1007/978-3-319-92330-7_9

9.1.1 Requirements

The design of the RADIO ecosystem architecture takes into account several requirements on the connectivity and availability of RADIO home deployments and the management of the sensitive data transmitted from and to the RADIO home deployments and the clinical sites.

The clinical sites connect and retrieve data from the RADIO home deployment. During connectivity loss, the RADIO home deployment should continue working autonomously and record data that can be later retrieved from the clinical site. However, RADIO home deployment should be able to transmit urgent notifications to the caregiver and clinical institution about the state of the deployment. In such a rare case, the RADIO ecosystem must be able to identify the disconnected home deployments and notify accordingly.

9.1.1.1 Privacy Requirements

The majority of the data produced by the RADIO home deployment are considered private, and certain privacy requirements must be taken into account in every layer of management (i.e., exchanging, retrieving, and processing).

Exchange of private data. Data exchange between RADIO home deployments and clinical institutes should be secured in the sense that no other party except the ones that are communicating can eavesdrop on the data exchanged. This fact includes parties from outside as well as from inside the RADIO ecosystem.

Management of private data. Clinical institute applications can retrieve private data only from the RADIO home deployments that have permission to do so. Moreover, different users of the clinical institute application must have different levels of clearance. The application should be able to validate a user's identity when user credentials are provided.

Processing of private data. Computations over data of all the RADIO home deployments can be defined in order to retrieve potentially useful statistical results for clinical experimentation. Those results should be presented to authorized researchers through the clinical experimentation application. However, the computations over the private data of the RADIO home deployments should be aggregated values and should not reveal individual data points of a known home deployment. In other words, one should be not able to distinguish either an individual data point or the initial RADIO home that has been retrieved from. Moreover, except the result produced, other parties of the RADIO ecosystem should not deduce (or gain access to) other parties of private data. The privacy-preserving processing will be discussed in more detail in Sect. 9.3.

9.2 The Architecture of the RADIO Ecosystem

In this section, we describe the architecture of the RADIO ecosystem and the interactions between its main entities and components.

9.2.1 Entities and Components

A *RADIO home deployment* is the main entity of the RADIO ecosystem. A RADIO home is essentially an appropriate setup space where the robot and the primary subject live and perform their daily activities. The RADIO home is a smart home in the sense that smart sensors and actuators are deployed in that space. A RADIO home can be, for example, a real house building or an appropriately configured room inside a health institution.

A *health institution* is an institution that provides care for the primary subjects and therefore has deployed several RADIO homes. A health institution, for instance, can be a hospital or a rehabilitation center. The medical personnel that monitor and provide care for a primary subject are considered to be the formal caregivers of that RADIO home and should have access to the clinical reports produced by the RADIO home deployment.

Apart from the formal caregivers, there exist the roles of the *informal caregiver* that are essentially people with no medical expertise but can be notified in case of an emergency that occurred in the RADIO home.

Last but not least, the *research centers* are also entities of the RADIO ecosystem. Those research centers are interested in conducting statistical analysis and data mining to the clinical data produced by the RADIO home deployments. The certified personnel that can analyze those data will be called health researchers.

RADIO home is the main data provider of the RADIO ecosystem. It processes the raw data retrieved from the deployed sensors and the robot and securely stores the processed data. The main components that reside in a RADIO home with respect to the other RADIO ecosystem components are as follows:

- *Sensing and Recognition System* that is the collection of sensors deployed in the RADIO home and in the robot, and the system of algorithms that can recognize abstract events from sensor measurements. This system produces the events that are stored in the "EventLog" database.
- *Actuation System* that is the collection of actuators in the RADIO home and in the robot that can perform actions in the physical world.
- *Smart Home Controller* that is responsible to integrate the sensor and actuation communication protocols (e.g., WiFi and Z-Wave) and dispatch measurements from sensors to the IoT platform and actuations from the IoT platform to the actuation system.

- *Medical Report Generator* that provides processed clinical data to the authorized personnel of the care institute in order to evaluate the condition and wellness of the subject.
- *Notification Generator* that provides alerts and notifications about urgent events occurring in the home to the registered caregivers and care institute personnel via the appropriate applications.
- *Privacy-Preserving Data Mining Component* that participates in and provides partial computations to a distributed computation initiated by the clinical experimentation application.

RADIO home deployments live and act inside the RADIO ecosystem. The RADIO home deployments integrate seamlessly in the RADIO ecosystem as nodes to an abstract network regardless of the different communication technologies and of the heterogeneous hardware and software components that comprise them.

9.2.2 Topology

Figure 9.1 presents an instance of a RADIO ecosystem network topology. In that topology, a collection of RADIO homes is logically organized as subsidiaries of a health institution. In the physical world, those RADIO homes can either reside in the health institution or be in a remote location. In either case, the health institution is considered to be connected to the RADIO home. The formal caregiver application is considered to be local to the health institution and can access the RADIO homes that are controlled by the health institute. The health researcher is using the clinical experimentation application to perform data analysis and be either located inside a dedicated research institute or inside the health institute.

We can distinguish the following communication channels:

- *Data Channel* that is the main channel of the network. This channel is used by the components of the ecosystem in order to provide or consume data. All the components must be able to connect to the data channel.
- *Notification Channel* that is the channel where the notifications flow. It is mainly used to provide notifications to the informal caregiver's application, and therefore, in principle, the only requirement is the connectivity between the informal caregiver's device and the corresponding RADIO home deployment.
- *Synchronization Channel* is the channel that connects the health institutions and the research centers of the ecosystem in order to synchronize their local registry data. It should be noted that in practice the data and the synchronization channels might share the same physical medium of transportation. However, conceptually there are two separate channels that have different connectivity requirements.

The organization of the RADIO ecosystem assumes that deployed RADIO homes must be associated with exactly one health institution. In other words,

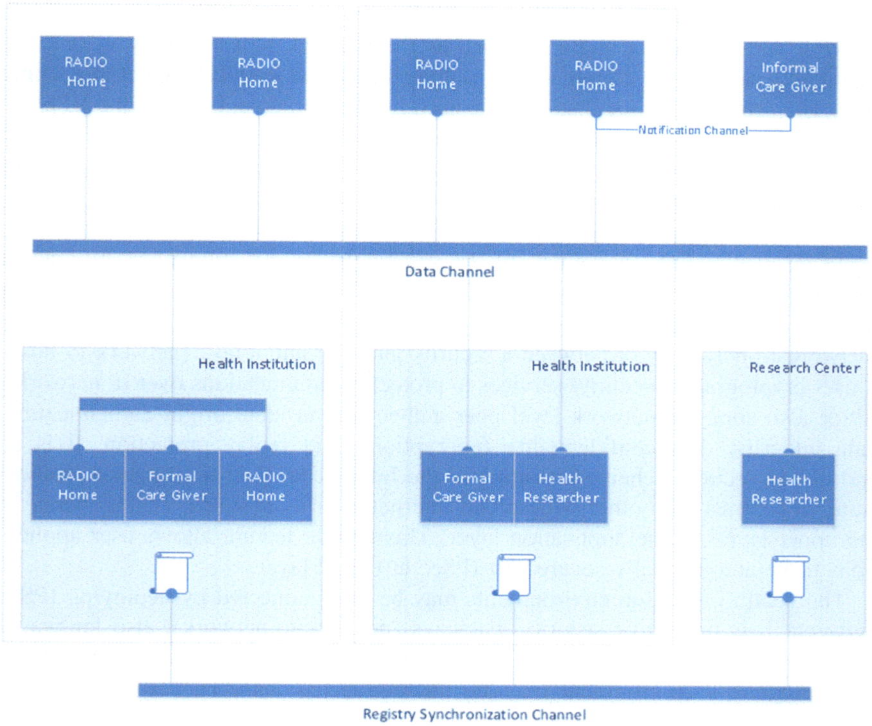

Fig. 9.1 The RADIO ecosystem network topology

RADIO homes cannot exist without an associated health institution that is most probably the institution which is affiliated with the formal caregiver.

The health institution also provides a discovery service to the other components of the RADIO ecosystem. More specifically, the care institution application and the clinical experimentation application can use the discovery service in order to locate the appropriate RADIO homes to contact. In order to provide that kind of service, the health institutes maintain a local registry of the registered RADIO homes. Each health institute synchronized its registry with the other health institutes in the RADIO ecosystem via the synchronization channel. This synchronization yields a global registry that can be used to discover components across the ecosystem.

9.2.3 *Security in Communication*

The overall communication architecture between the caregiver's environment and the health institution environment, as well as between the health institution environments themselves has to take into account the sensitivity of personal data that must be exchanged between the above-mentioned entities.

The use of Virtual Private Network (VPN) technology, which extends a private network across a public network, such as the Internet, is a necessity in order to seamlessly achieve the communication objectives of the RADIO project in a secure way. The proposed protocol suite to be used for the implementation of the VPNs in the RADIO project is the Internet Protocol Security (IPSec).

IPSec is an open standard protocol suite for secure Internet protocol (IP) communications by authenticating and encrypting each IP packet of a communication session. IPSec includes protocols for establishing mutual authentication between agents at the beginning of the session and negotiation of cryptographic keys to be used during the session. IPSec can be used in protecting data flows between a pair of hosts (host-to-host), between a pair of security gateways (network-to-network), or between a security gateway and a host (network-to-host). It uses cryptographic security services to protect communications over IP networks. IPSec also supports network-level peer authentication, data origin authentication, data integrity, data confidentiality (encryption), and replay protection. It is an end-to-end security scheme operating in the Internet layer of the Internet protocol suite, in contrast with other widespread Internet security systems, which operate in the upper layers at the application layer. This unique feature allows user applications to be automatically secured by IPSec at the IP layer.

The health institution environments may be interconnected by deploying IPSec between their respective security gateways (network-to-network), also known as site-to-site IPSec VPN, by means of either a partial mesh or a full mesh topology. The caregiver's environment may be interconnected with the respective health institution by deploying IPSec between the security gateway of the health institution and the workstation and/or mobile device of the caregiver's environment (network-to-host), also known as remote access IPSec VPN, by means of a hub and spoke topology where the health institutions are considered hubs and the caregiver's environments spokes. In either case, a secure IPSec tunnel, which provides the secure transmission of sensitive personal data in a transparent to the application way, is created between the respective endpoints.

The deployment of IPSec VPNs between the RADIO project entities, which need to exchange sensitive data, is a scalable standardized solution that builds secure data channels on top of the Internet which is considered an "untrusted" network. The overall design allows also the creation of multiple connections (using site-to-site VPNs or remote access VPNs) between entities, which provide a level of redundancy in case of communication network failures. The "extension" of the several private networks over the VPN connections facilitates the overall network monitoring of the various devices that are located in disparate networks.

9.2.4 Changes in the Topology

During the lifecycle of the RADIO ecosystem, it is natural to expect that RADIO homes will be deployed or removed from the ecosystem, and health institutes and research centers will join. We distinguish three different procedures that must be followed when a new site is added to the topology.

Assume first the deployment of a new RADIO home. As mentioned previously, each RADIO home is affiliated with a health institution.

1. After the installation of the physical devices (e.g., Smart home sensors, RADIO robot) in the RADIO home, the RADIO home (specifically the smart home controller) is registered to the IoT platform. This includes the deployment of a signed digital certificate.
2. The health institution registers the newly deployed RADIO home to its local registry. The registration procedure produces VPN credentials for the RADIO home that are transferred in a secure and off-band way and deployed in the RADIO home in order to establish a secure connection with the affiliated health institution.
3. Authorization and authentication of the appropriate medical personnel are defined by the administrator of the health institution.
4. Informal caregivers that will be notified for urgent events are also defined for the specific RADIO home.

Assume now that the health institution decides to join the ecosystem. This requires the following steps:

1. Deploy the site-to-site VPN with other health institutions that require a valid signed digital certificate.
2. Install the registry component and initiate the first synchronization with the rest of the health institutions. This requires to know at least one institution or research center that has already joined the RADIO ecosystem.
3. Start deploying the RADIO homes following the steps described previously.

Lastly, the procedure for a research center is similar to the health institution with the difference that the registry is read only. More specifically, the procedure comprises the following steps:

1. Deploy the site-to-site VPN with other health institutions that require a valid signed digital certificate.
2. Install the registry component and initiate the first synchronization with the rest of the health institutions. This requires to know at least one institution or research center that has already joined the RADIO ecosystem.
3. Define the researchers that are authorized to access the data analysis module of the RADIO ecosystem.

9.3 Remote Medical Assessment

The formal caregivers of the RADIO ecosystem must have access to the recorded data of their assigned subjects for health monitoring reasons. In contrast to the health researchers, the formal caregivers are interested in a more detailed and focused report about the activities of their assigned subjects.

The events that occur in a RADIO home are recorded in a database and can be accessed by the formal caregiver's frontend. Each database corresponds to a specific RADIO home (and, by extension, to a specific subject). The nature of the recorded data nominates the time-series database management system as the predominant choice for using the RADIO ecosystem. More specifically, InfluxDB, an open-source time-series database, is used as the backend of the RADIO ecosystem data management.

The schema of each database consists of multiple time series that contain the following information:

- *Time* of the occurred event.
- *Participant* an alphanumeric identifier used as a field key to identify the subject of the event. This is mainly used for visualization and reporting reasons. Since each database corresponds to a single SubjectID, the field is expected to be constant throughout the time series. However, the existence of this field helps during the reporting of multiple subjects.
- *Measurement* is a field value that contains the measured quantity of the event. The measurement type and value range depend on the type of the event.

The recorded events include

- chair transfer;
- bed transfer;
- four-meter walk;
- pill intake;
- TV watching;
- meal preparation; and
- going out of the room.

The events are visualized as graphs and tables. The visualization tool used in our case is Grafana, an open-source user interface focused on visualizing time series in various ways.

Figure 9.2 depicts an overview of the visualizations implemented for the formal caregiver's data access. The events that contain measurable quantities (chair transfer time, bed transfer time, and time to walk 4 m) are depicted as line graphs over time, while the other events are depicted as tables.

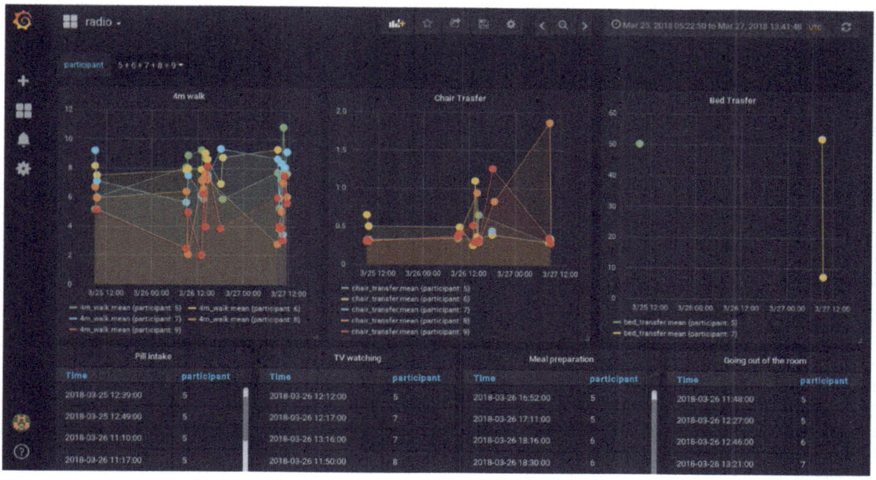

Fig. 9.2 An overview of visualizations provided to the medical assessment personnel

9.4 Privacy-Preserving Statistical Analysis

The insights gained by the large-scale analysis of health-related data can have an enormous impact in public health and medical research, but access to such personal and sensitive data poses serious privacy implications for the data provider and a heavy data security and administrative burden on the data consumer. The discussion on what exactly it means to not disclose private data [1] and the discussion on policies for balancing between scientific advancement and privacy [2] are very relevant but should be complemented by the equally relevant discussion of whether there is tension at all between data privacy and data-driven research. In other words, it is not straightforward if private data can be insulated from medical research workflows without compromising either.

As anonymization has been repeatedly proven to be inadequate [3], attention has turned to research in cryptography and distributed computation. These fields can provide methods for computing aggregates and statistics without revealing the specific data values involved in the computation, offering a much stronger guarantee of privacy than anonymization. However, from the perspective of the data mining practitioners and the medical researchers, there is still a residue of functionality missing between their workflows over anonymized data and what is technically possible to achieve without accessing specific data points.

The RADIO ecosystem architecture foresees the statistical analysis of the data produced by the RADIO home deployments in a way that no requirements are violated. In particular, a health researcher should be able to use the clinical experimentation application in order to pose statistical queries against the collection of the data that reside in the RADIO ecosystem. However, the data produced in each RADIO home deployment are considered private, and as such the privacy-preserving data mining (PPDM) component must respect the privacy requirements for managing and processing such data.

The proposed architectural approach is reduced into two main ideas:

- The set of the valid statistical queries that are allowed by the system must be appropriately restricted in order to avoid exposing individual data points but only aggregated data. A wide range of existing statistical method depends only on aggregation of data, and therefore can also be formalized in that restricted query set.
- Instead of fetching raw data in order to compute the aggregation, the computations will be performed local to the data and only the result will be transmitted. In order words, the RADIO home deployment will contain the processing units in order to perform partial computations on its private data. Moreover, multiple RADIO homes must collaborate in such a way that can produce the final result of the computation and at the same time will not expose any of their private data points.

The scope of our discussion here is restricted to the data and processing required to empirically validate an already formulated hypothesis over a larger dataset than what can reasonably be made available to research. Naturally, part of the researchers' workflow involves browsing data in order to formulate a hypothesis. This initial hypothesis formulation remains in the scope of smaller experimental data specifically collected and licensed to be shared.

The system architecture can be perceived as a stack of three layers, and each layer depends on the functionality provided from the layer at the lower stage. The upper layer, called the Medical Researcher's interface, accepts from the medical researcher the method with the initial parameters to be executed by the system. The purpose of this interface is to provide a familiar environment to the researcher, and therefore in our current implementation this layer is developed in the R language. The initial parameters are transformed appropriately in order to be passed to the next layer, which is the compilation layer. At that stage, the high-level parameters and commands of the statistical method are transformed into low-level instruction for accessing the private databases of the agents. An instruction represents an aggregation over a selection of data. Currently, the aggregation operation is summation. However, the aggregations that are both feasible by the system and safe for preserving privacy depend on the secure protocol used. These instructions will be eventually evaluated by the lowest layer of the architecture, the privacy protocol layer. Figure 9.2 depicts the system architecture and the information exchanged between the layers.

9.4.1 The Compilation Layer

This layer is responsible for the communication between the two other layers. Specifically, it translates the arguments of the secure statistic to a suitable format, and thus it defines the appropriate data that are going to be used for the statistic computation. Moreover, it converts the simple statistic equations to a set of summations, a compatible format to achieve the secure summation protocol. Therefore, a set of instructions is composed where each instruction represents a summation equation of the statistic with the appropriate parameter's set for its computation. During the execution, the compilation layer gives the privacy protocol layer a single instruction at a time and it receives its result. After the execution of the whole set, it computes the statistic and the analysis parameters. The statistic result is sent back to the Medical Researcher's interface layer.

9.4.2 The Aggregation Protocol

This layer executes the privacy protocol between the AAL agents. To deal with the concurrent computation of each instruction, we model our agents as actors. Each actor makes the appropriate computations with respect to the given instruction and its private data. These computations can easily be done since every AAL agent controls its corresponding health records. After the computation of the value, which represents the initial secret, the privacy protocol is executed. The protocol may involve all the actors to work collaboratively in order to compute the aggregation of their secrets without revealing the actual secrets to each other or the agent requesting the aggregation. The aggregated result is collected a designated actor. The selection of such actor is irrelevant and can be done randomly.

9.4.3 Discussion

The proposed system architecture assumes that

- the statistical analysis that is to be carried out can be implemented using the set of aggregation instructions provided by the aggregation protocol. In other words, the algorithm should not depend on individual data points.
- a summation protocol exists that guarantees privacy.

The first assumption holds, since the most commonly used class of data mining algorithms can be expressed as an iteration of summation expressions [4]. If needed, categorical operators can be implemented based on summation [5]. Regarding the second assumption, we will now proceed to discuss the summation protocols that can be used in our architecture.

Most of the related studies guarantee their privacy by utilizing encryption or differential privacy techniques. These approaches do not fit in our problem, because we deal with medical history data that are distributed across AAL agents. In homomorphic techniques, a master agent shares a public key with the rest of the agents, in order to encrypt their data, and keeps a private key for the final decryption. Such a mechanism is privately weak in the case of collaborative computations, because if the medical researcher (master agent) and one AAL agent collude, they can learn another AAL agent's private value. This makes the technical protocol weak, as it places a heavy burden on non-technical policies and protocols to guarantee the integrity of the medical researcher. Since our main aim is to alleviate the need for non-technical policies and protocols and to make it easier for medical researchers to run statistics over data point, they are not meant to access directly, and homomorphism encryption does not cover our requirements.

In addition, differential privacy is also not applicable, from both the perspective of the medical researcher and from that of the AAL agent. From the perspective of the medical researcher, differential privacy computes approximations. From the perspective of the AAL agent, the secret value can be approximated by its repeated querying, since a different perturbation of the real secret needs to be computed for each query. The AAL agent cannot produce a single perturbed value and use this for all queries, since it needs to be re-computed to follow the distribution parameters requested by the medical researcher. This might be less of a problem in time-series data (such as power grid data or traffic data) but can result in substantial information leaking in static historical data, such as health records.

9.4.4 The RASSP Protocol

The RADIO data mining system is unaware of the underlying privacy-preserving protocol that it is using. In this section, we will present the RASSP (RADIO Secure Summation Protocol) that satisfies the requirements needed by the system to ensure privacy preservation.

Secret sharing schemes divide a secret into many shares which can be distributed to n mutually suspicious agents. The initial secret can be revealed if any k of these n agents combine their shares. We will call such schemes as *(k, n)*-threshold schemes. If such a scheme also possesses the homomorphism property, then multiple secrets can be combined by direct computation only on the shares. Such schemes are usually called composite secret sharing schemes [6].

More specifically, assume n mutually suspicious agents and each agent holds a secret s_i. The desired computation is combined into a super-secret s under an operation $\oplus$. Using a secret sharing scheme, each s_i can be split into k shares d_{i1}, …, d_{ik} such that given a known function F_I it is the case that $s_i = F_I(d_{i1}, \ldots, d_{ik})$. The composition of the shares d_1, d_1' yields a *super-share* $d_1 \otimes d_1'$. In other words, the ($\oplus$, $\otimes$)-homomorphism property implies that the compositions of the shares under the operator $\otimes$ are shares of the composition under the operator $\oplus$.

Overall, the advantage of having a composite secret sharing scheme is that secret cannot be obtained, only if k or more agents collude and combine their sub-shares. In addition, this protocol is suitable to our approach from the AAL agent's point of view, because it does not use a trusted third party or depends on cryptographic assumptions, while at the same time it is *k*-secure. This approach represents a secure summation protocol that can easily be applied to collaborative agent systems. Based on this mathematical foundation, we will now proceed to present the RASSP protocol, a $(\oplus, \otimes)$-homomorphic composite secret sharing scheme.

Figure 9.3 gives an example of the above description for a system of three AAL agents. In this example, *House1* has the private value v_1 and produces three numbers: r_{11}, r_{12}, and r_{13}. Then, it shares r_{12} and r_{13} with *House2* and *House3*, keeping r_{11} hidden. *House1* receives two numbers (r_{21}, r_{31}) from the other AAL agents. It then shares the computed Y_1, so that F_I can be computed by summing all Y_i. $F_I(Y_1, Y_2, Y_3)$ computes the sum of all three AAL agents' secret values (Fig. 9.4).

The described secure summation protocol is suitable for computing medical statistics and preserves privacy at the same time. The only constraint is that the resulted outcome is a sum of the private values, and thus the statistic equations should be converted into a summation form. The summation form results in accurate values and not approximations, while simultaneously it can easily be

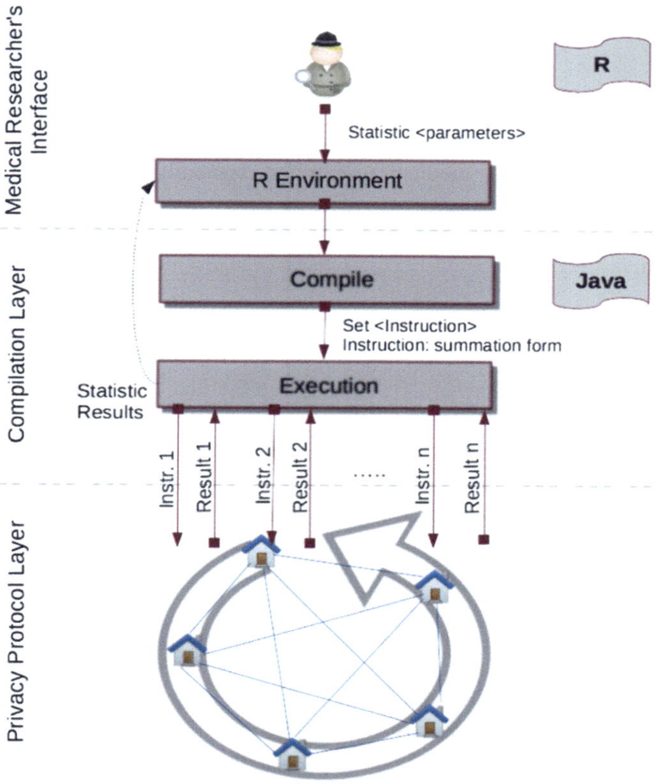

Fig. 9.3 The system architecture and the information exchanged between the layers

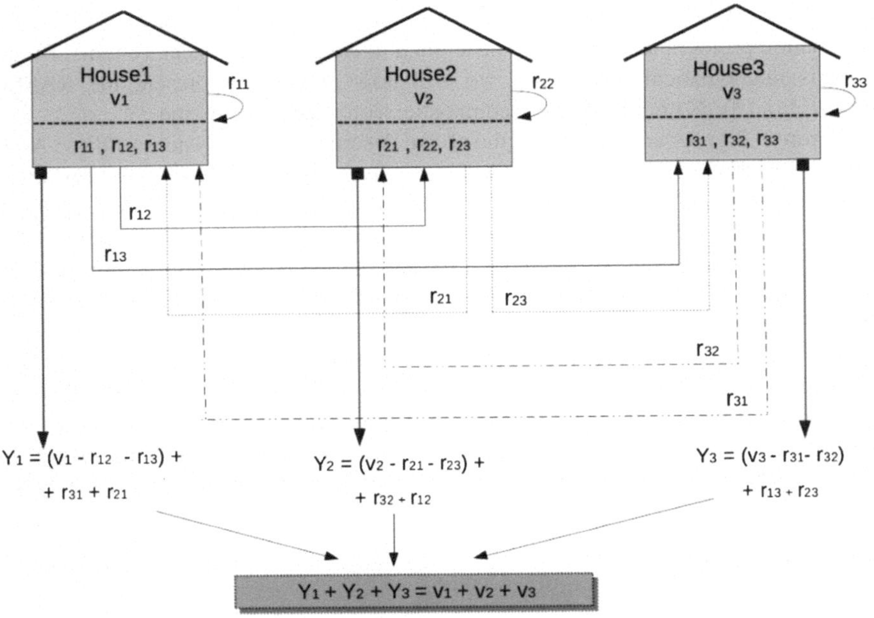

Fig. 9.4 An example of the RASSP protocol

parallelized [7]. Besides, medical researchers typically use descriptive statistics which utilize numerical descriptors such as mean and standard deviation. These descriptors can easily be converted into a summation form and thus computed by our system.

9.5 Conclusions

RADIO proved the concept of connecting RADIO homes and medical institutions into the RADIO ecosystem, adding value to the health data collected by RADIO homes by making it available not only for medical monitoring but also for medical research. Specifically, RADIO developed network security and access control guidelines for direct access to health data by the competent medical personnel, as well as the RASSP protocol for the privacy-preserving mining of the data collected in each home's database. These expose appropriate programmatic interfaces, so that, and depending on one's access and use case, individual data and time series can be visualized to monitor particular end users and statistical data aggregations can be visualized or used by R programs to carry out medical research.

The RADIO ecosystem is a central part of the overall solution offered in particular in light of the future project exploitation and commercialization, as it touches upon uptake by medical institutions and public bodies. The most innovative outcome is the ability to serve sensitive health data to medical research without compromising privacy.

References

1. Clifton, C., Kantarcioglu, M., & Vaidya, J. (2002). Defining privacy for data mining. *National Science Foundation Workshop on Next Generation Data Mining, 1*(26).
2. Horvitz, E., & Mulligan, D. (2015). Data, privacy, and the greater good. *Science, 349*(6245), 253–255.
3. Ohm, P. (2009). Broken promises of privacy: Responding to the surprising failure of anonymization. *UCLA Law Review, 57,* 1701.
4. Kearns, M. (1998). Efficient noise-tolerant learning from statistical queries. *Journal of the ACM (JACM), 45*(6), 983–1006.
5. Kissner, L., & Song, D. (2005). Privacy-preserving set operations. In *Annual International Cryptology Conference*. Berlin: Springer.
6. Benaloh, J. C. (1986). Secret sharing homomorphisms: Keeping shares of a secret secret. In *Conference on the Theory and Application of Cryptographic Techniques*. Berlin: Springer.
7. Chu, C.-T., Kim, S. K., Lin, Y.-A., Yu, Y. Y., Bradski, G., Ng, A. Y., et al. (2007). Map-reduce for machine learning on multicore. *Advances in Neural Information Processing Systems*.

Part III
The Road to Commercialization

Chapter 10
Roadmap to Expanding Alternatives to Hospitalization

Roberta Annicchiarico, Fulvia Adriano, Sergio Ariño-Blasco and Diana Navarro-Llobet

10.1 Aging Society

Elderly population is growing faster than all younger age groups. The most recent data on global aging report that the number of persons aged 60 years or older is expected to more than double by 2050 and to more than triple by 2100, rising from 962 million globally in 2017 to 2.1 billion in 2050 and 3.1 billion in 2100 [1]. According to United Nations, it is estimated that virtually every country in the world is experiencing growth in the number and proportion of older persons in their population. As a consequence of this, population aging is becoming one of the most significant social phenomena of the twenty-first century, leading to repercussions for several sectors of society, mainly the demand for goods and services and implications for labor and financial markets. When particularly looking at European Union, on January 2016, the whole population was estimated at 510.3 million; while people up to 14 years were 15.6%, elderly (65 years old or over) were 19.2%. Notably, such an increase is of 0.3% compared with the previous year and even of 2.4% when compared with 10 years earlier. According to recent statistics [2], across the EU member states, the lowest share of young people is recorded in

R. Annicchiarico (✉) · F. Adriano
Clinical and Behavioral Neurology Laboratory, IRCCS Fondazione Santa Lucia, via Ardeatina 306, 00179 Rome, Italy
e-mail: r.annicchiarico@hsantalucia.it

F. Adriano
e-mail: f.adriano@hsantalucia.it

S. Ariño-Blasco · D. Navarro-Llobet
Hospital General de Granollers, Av. Francesc Ribas, S/N, 08402 Granollers, Spain
e-mail: sarino@fhag.es

D. Navarro-Llobet
e-mail: diananavarro@fhag.es

V. Karkaletsis et al. (eds.), *RADIO–Robots in Assisted Living*,
https://doi.org/10.1007/978-3-319-92330-7_10

Germany (13.2%) and about the share of persons aged 65 or older, the highest shares were in Italy (22%), Greece (21.3%), and Germany (21.1%).

Although it is widely recognized that new generations of elderly are relatively active and healthy when compared with past generations of older people, however, it is undeniable that aging process naturally leads to an increase of frailty and vulnerability. Indeed, compared to younger populations, older adults are more vulnerable to multimorbidity and chronic illnesses, and thus it is estimated that 50% of hospitalized adults are 65 years or older and this proportion is only expected to increase [3, 4].

10.2 Elderly Services

As a consequence of the abovementioned demographic and societal developments, health and social care systems are asked to face a growing demand for services and goods for elderly population. For example, demand for long-term care (LTC) services is expected to increase in the next decades. Particularly, projections of LTC expenditures showed that home care is in high demand. Although it is a matter of common knowledge that European citizens prefer to live and, if possible, spend their final days at home, however, public policy has been slow, and still is, to support a shift from institutions and hospitals to home-based care settings [5]. Nevertheless, all over Europe, a major share of the older population in need of care is receiving care from informal carers (e.g., spouses, children, and other family members), even in those countries having large publicly supported elderly care services [6]. Moreover, it is reported that most public funding for LTC services goes to institutional services [5], even over 70% in Belgium, Iceland, and Switzerland. Impressively, such funding accounts for 0.3–3.9% of gross domestic product. At the same time, LTC institutions often require, on top of public funding, high fees to the users and their relatives, and these in some cases exceed the net monthly salary of an average production worker.

Accurate forecast analyses are performed by decision-makers who expect homes to be a cheaper alternative to hospital-based services and nursing home care [7]. Nevertheless, at present in most European countries, demand for home care cannot yet be met by the available formal home care schemes, and therefore it is needed that policy-makers will look for inspiration beyond the usual models and good practices to find solutions in response to these challenges.

10.3 Long-Term Care Services for Elderly in Europe

World Health Organization defines LTC as "the system of activities undertaken by informal caregivers (family, friends, and/or neighbours) and/or professionals (health and social services) to ensure that a person who is not fully capable of self-care can maintain the highest possible quality of life, according to his or her individual preferences, with the greatest possible degree of independence, autonomy, participation, personal fulfilment and human dignity" [8]. When talking about elderly population, by informal caregivers, it is meant family, in-home nurses, friends, and neighbors; by professionals, it is meant health and social services provided by public health, primary care, home care and rehabilitation services, palliative care, and institutional care in nursing homes and hospices.

The way health systems respond to the need of LTC of elderly is strictly related to the local health service organization. In each European country, national health systems provide care coverage mainly on the basis of their respective past tradition [9, 10]. Indeed, national health systems of European countries are based on elements from the Beveridgean and Bismarckian model systems together with conservative and family traditions. Particularly, the Bismarckian model views LTC protection (as well as any social insurance) as depending on labor and social contributions. Therefore, insurance helps contributors with proportionality of benefits to contributions. This model is mainly adopted in Germany, Denmark, and the Netherlands. On the contrary, in countries adopting the Beveridgean model (also called "social democratic model") such as Sweden and Spain, social protection is supported by the national government that decentralizes implementation to municipalities. This system is financed by taxes and is unrelated to employment, thus striving for egalitarianism through uniform benefits. A special case is the Anglo-Saxon model, adopted in the United Kingdom and Ireland where healthcare is provided through a national tax-supported system, although most recently supplementary services, partially covered by private health insurance, have been gaining in importance. This model is also known as "liberal", due to its liberal attitude to markets. Indeed, most of the funds are used for the working-age population, and less for pensioners. Moreover, it is previous employment that defines the access to benefits, thus resulting in that those who have not been employed would not be admitted to such benefits and this might constitute a problem for those family members who have to stay at home to take care of their disabled and/or elderly relatives.

Overall, the use of LTC services by elderly varies widely across European countries. The share of elderly receiving services in institutions ranges from less than 1% in Poland and Russian Federation to 9% in Iceland. As for those receiving publicly funded services at home, the share ranges from very small in many countries in Eastern Europe to 25% in Denmark [5]. Finally, about Southern Europe countries, according to Bocquaire [9], the traditional model tends to leave LTC responsibilities on families, although this is progressively challenged with rising rates of female employment.

Below is reported, regardless of the models specifically adopted in the individual countries, the main LTC solutions adopted across European countries.

Home Care is a service carried out in the home of the elderly. Usually, it is targeted to older people recently released by the hospital or in need of regular treatments, with the aim of supporting them in daily living, thus allowing them to continue to live in their own homes for longer and avoiding inappropriate hospital admissions. Home care services are provided by three different kinds of persons/ entities: (i) Integrated home care services. Integrated and coordinated health and social activities have been accredited for this function. Health services are medical care (geriatricians, psychiatrists, etc.), nursing, rehabilitation, medicines, and prosthesis supply services; social services are personal care, meals, housework, laundry, and administrative services. Such services may also be provided by public sector but the law on eligibility for accessing them often covers only persons without adequate family support, who are dependent on the help of another person, and poor. Moreover, funding remains a long-term problem and its consequences are non-permanent work contracts for staff, non-payment of salaries, and long-term insecurity; (ii) In-home nurses. These are mainly migrant women and it is estimated that many (especially those providing a 24 h/service) are without work permits, without social insurance, without residence permits, and, at least initially, they are usually paid around the lowest basic salary; (iii) Family and friends networks. When it comes to the need for care for loved ones, the family and friends' networks choose to be involved in this. Although this is often due to the limited welfare state provision, however, this is also related to traditional ways. Indeed, it is expected that older people, who have contributed throughout their lives to the practical and financial support of children and grandchildren, can draw on the same network when they need help. On the other side, often there are no services for the carers (e.g., psychosocial support) and no financial support is provided for those who are sometimes forced to quit their jobs in order to assist their relatives. Differently, in some other cases, a reimbursement is offered for those persons needing such services. For example, an LTC insurance was established by the German welfare state in 1996 to either provide elderly the care services they need or cash benefits to pay for a private caregiver, such as a family member.

Day Centers are (mainly local) semi-residential structures hosting elderly people. They are usually open during the day (less frequently, some semi-institutional care services are open during the night). They provide healthcare (e.g., prevention, therapy, and rehabilitation) and social care services (e.g., personal care and promotion of personal autonomy, entertainment, job therapy, and social activities). Furtherly, possible additional formal care services are provided through the accommodation of elderly in residential apartments, in sheltered housing, and under foster care.

Residential structures are nursing homes which provide health and social care, and functional rehabilitation for elderly people presenting disabilities. The staff is made of physicians, nurses, social workers, and psychologists. Such structures can offer two kinds of care, extensive or intensive: the first comprising long-term rehabilitation and accommodation through hospitalization; the latter includes rehabilitation with high medical importance but it might also provide hospice and palliative care for terminal patients. Residential structures can also offer institutional care, an LTC service adapted to the type and degree of dependency, and the intensity of care required by the user (i.e., on a permanent basis, when the residential center becomes the user's usual residence, or temporarily, when the person requires a stay for the purpose of convalescence, during holiday periods, or at weekends). Residential structures, when publicly financed, have a limited access, often with long waiting lists, and are mainly addressed to the poor. Otherwise, private organizations and licensed individuals offer a variety of health- and care-related services for a negotiable fee through private hospitals, clinics, and residential structures. These are usually monitored by a public body, e.g., the corresponding prefecture.

Private not-for-profit sector. This sector deserves a particular mention as, by means of non-governmental organizations, charity and philanthropic organizations, churches and privately funded foundations, many services and programs are offered. They are monitored and regulated by public bodies to assure both the legality and quality of services they provide and staff is composed of paid employees in cooperation with volunteers. In many countries, these services cover the inadequacies of the welfare system and they are partners of the state in the provision of some social services.

10.4 New Frontiers in LTC for Elderly: ICT Services

With the elderly population growing faster than any other, an appropriate social and financial plan for LTC targeted to elderly is needed and it should aim at balancing between informal care and public support and services. A sustainable LTC system might be based on a proper combination of public health and social services, supported informal care, and technical aids.

With regard to technical aids, the demand for ICT products and services supporting elderly population in their daily living is enormously growing, yet is still characterized by

- *high fragmentation*: the available products and services are still characterized by high heterogeneity and poor standardization at the European level. As a consequence, there is a lack of a wide and systematized diffusion of such products and services;
- *inelasticity*: the lack of close substitutes for ICT products and services causes a weak price elasticity;
- *scarcity*: in spite the growing demand, not all elderly actually can access assistive ICT devices and services; and
- *need of adaptation*: several products need to be adapted to the specific characteristics and needs of users.

Overall, although a growing number of products aiming at supporting and enhancing daily living of elderly people are currently available in the market, however, often they can address a limited target of users and only provide partial and/or superficial solutions.

The current scenario in European countries seems to show a co-existence of services different in terms of “delivery”, thus resulting in a sharp separation between healthcare and social care and their corresponding ICT services, often named *telecare* (i.e., social alarms) and *telehealth*. The differentiation between what is funded under LTC insurance furtherly confirms this traditional separation, for example, social alarms (i.e., telecare) are basically covered, while home telehealth often is not and is just beginning to be covered in some countries (e.g., Germany). Therefore, the first urgent need is developing integrated models of social and health cares, and thus only later properly integrated ICT services can be implemented. With the increasing average age of European population, a growing number of people will develop chronic diseases, thus potentially needing both telecare and home healthcare services.

10.5 Vision and Objectives

The demographic and epidemiological transition has taken us to the crossroads of aging and chronic diseases, forcing a diversification in the provision of care. Healthcare policies constantly try to adapt to the demographic and epidemiological needs of our society, and nowadays must be submitted under the prism of "the triple aim": better health system, better health, and lower cost [11].

Healthcare policies force to rethink models that cover the increasingly complex needs of elderly groups, considering integrated social and health models instead of fragmented care [12]. Obviously, it is about implementing the most effective and efficient models, based on scientific evidence; unfortunately, this is scarce in our field [13].

Despite the moment of rapid technological development in which we live, there are still many questions left unanswered, many referents to the field of aging. We must not only deal with the impact on the level of independence achieved with the intervention but also if the needs of the elderly have been considered in their design. Still today, we have challenges ahead in the design and evaluation of intervention studies with new technologies. The focus has mainly been on studies of satisfaction and feasibility rather than in studies of effectiveness and cost-effectiveness. An extra challenge in gerontechnology research is that of implementation and adherence to interventions, showing low rates of achievement [14–16]. These circumstances show the relevance of our research, which pretends to easy access to relevant technologies.

The plan of the consortium from a clinical point of view is focused on improving access to RADIO in order to improve quality of home and community care for seniors. From a medical perspective, the system could help in two ways: to primary users (prevention and wellness services, for education and lifestyle changes, and for family caregivers) or to the healthcare setting (home care, nursing home, and rehabilitation) with a large amount of benefits for different end users.

By using RADIO system, clinicians can easily monitor "risk situations" and early detect clinical problems both improving patient's quality of life and reducing caregiver's burden. Healthcare facilities providing services to elderly can improve the quality of provided assistance as well. Next, we list most relevant areas of interest in which the system may be used and integrated into the future management of the elderly patient from the medical perspective.

10.6 Prevention and Wellness Services

Prevention activities seek to avoid the onset of disease, detect the onset of disease early through screening, and stop disease from progressing or worsening. Prevention in elderly people includes and has to be focused on prevention of frailty and disability. Screening and early detection refer to a broad range of instruments—including exams, tests, and clinical guidelines—used to identify a disease in individuals who do not have symptoms. While not all screenings have proven effective, employing evidence-based detection techniques has the potential to improve health outcomes and lower the cost of treatment by detecting and mitigating the progression of numerous diseases associated with aging, including multiple forms of cancer, cardiovascular disease, chronic kidney disease, diabetes, hepatitis, as well as Alzheimer's, dementia, depression, and alcohol abuse.

Screening and early detection are especially crucial in a frail elderly. Frailty is one of the most relevant geriatric conditions, which has shown to be extremely suitable to serve as target for preventive and therapeutic interventions. However, other geriatric conditions such as functional impairment and dementia are frequently unrecognized or inadequately addressed in older adults. For many elderly individuals, the loss of everyday competence may stem from a variety of sources; notable among these is the presence of disease. Often these problems arise gradually and may not even be considered a problem for some time.

The RADIO system can help caregiver in the management of their relatives. The system can detect any possible change from the iADL standard pattern and alert caregivers and physicians. In other terms, an alert can be sent if, in the daily routine, something is not happening as usual (e.g., user has not taken his pills, user has reduced his weekly physical activity, etc.).

10.7 Home Care Solutions

Together, ICT and domotics may deeply influence the rise of new models of care through the connections among professionals, the changing roles of formal and informal actors and of the patients, the reduction of the functional limitations and the frailness, and the reduction of the burden for informal carers. Overall, the increasing synergy between the ICT and the home-based advanced equipment—which can be expected to grow further in the next years—may reach the effect of enabling effective and innovative care models, thus facilitating the management of deep changes in the care organization and in the respective roles of all the formal and informal actors (including the beneficiary) [17].

10.8 Residential Care Solutions

Ambient-assisted living (AAL) technologies aim to assist elderly people and their caregivers using a set of technologies (such as sensors, actuators, interaction devices, and, more recently, robots) in order to respond specific patient's needs. Nursing home providers can also improve efficacy and efficiency [18] using these technologies.

One of the goals of the technology is to ensure greater safety. In this sense, the most rewarding areas according to the elderly are fall detection [19]. However, activity monitoring, iADL as well as ADL, could have an important role as detection method for early diagnosis [20]. Similarly, one of the major potential utilities of the technology is having an accurate way of performing human activity patterns such ADL-iADL assessments, somehow "equivalent to healthcare professional's assessment". Functional assessment is a very time-consuming exercise in everyday practice and any robust and ergonomic improvement will be very much appreciated.

10.9 Rehabilitative Solutions

For the older patient, the discharge from a hospital is a critical issue, when decisions are made that may influence the rest of that person's life. Discharge planning is a challenging task under the best of circumstances, and changes in the healthcare environment have made it almost impossible to do such planning well. Even under the best of circumstances, the discharge planning process in hospitals is inherently complex. Information from many sources must be gathered, including patient-specific information regarding functional status and patient and family preferences, as well as information about available community resources. With shortened lengths of hospital stay, it is difficult to assess a patient's medical prognosis and pre-hospital level of functioning, much less predict post-hospital potential. Effective discharge planning can decrease the chances that a patient is readmitted to a hospital, help in recovery, ensure medications are prescribed and given correctly, and adequately prepare caregivers to take care of their relatives. Key elements of a well-managed post-hospital discharge geriatric assessment include targeting criteria to identify vulnerable patients, a program of multidimensional assessment, comprehensive discharge planning, and home follow-up.

Efforts to re-engineer the discharge process to assure a safe transition involve such issues as improved clinician communication, patient education, information technology systems, involvement of community-based providers, and arrangements for prompt follow-up [21]. Such interventions have the potential to substantially improve patient care and reduce healthcare expenditures. The patient's assessment before discharge and the follow-up program are identified as the two characteristics necessary in a formally structured discharge planning program for effective care of older patients [22]. RADIO system can provide a comprehensive assessment before and after the discharge to home or to nursing home.

10.10 Conclusions

It seems possible to affirm that in the healthcare sector there are many possibilities to integrate RADIO system with a large amount of benefits for different end users. In fact, RADIO system can improve elderly and/or patients quality of life. Caregivers may obtain many benefits as well, as their care burden would result significantly reduced. By using RADIO system, clinicians can easily monitor "risk situations" and early detect clinical problems. Finally, healthcare facilities providing services to elderly can improve quality of provided assistance.

The plan of the consortium from the clinical point of view is focused on improving access to RADIO system in order to improve quality of home and community care for seniors. It will help seniors to live independently in their own homes and communities, avoiding social isolation and loneliness. It will reduce pressure on family members—many of whom are already balancing full-time employment and parenting their own children—to act as care providers. It is also the most cost-effective way to increase access to hospital services for people of all ages.

Assessment of function and targeting interventions during hospitalization are critically important to acute care of older adults. The impact of functional decline on resource utilization and healthcare costs may further reinforce the need to assess and intervene to prevent functional decline. In literature, among health providers and within governments, there is growing recognition that a comprehensive and well-coordinated home and community care system can significantly alleviate pressure in the most expensive part of the health system—hospitals—by reducing wait times for both emergency and surgical services.

On the other hand, the real strength of ICT lies in the opportunity to combine and analyze data from various sources. ICT is also strong in collecting and storing data over long periods of time: significant but not obvious changes in one's health status can be detected and signaled by continuous analysis of such data as done by RADIO system.

References

1. United Nations, Department of Economic and Social Affairs, Population Division. (2017). *World population prospects: The 2017 revision, key findings and advance tables*. Working Paper No. ESA/P/WP/248.
2. Eurostat Statistics Explained. (2017). *Population structure and ageing*. http://ec.europa.eu/eurostat/statistics-explained/index.php/Population_structure_and_ageing. Accessed March 15, 2018.

3. Bell, S. P., & Saraf, A. A. (2016). Epidemiology of multimorbidity in older adults with cardiovascular disease. *Clinics in Geriatric Medicine, 32*(2), 215–226.
4. Bergvalle, D., Charbit, C., Kraan, D., & Merk, O. (2006). Intergovernmental transfers and decentralised public spending. *OECD Journal on Budgeting, 5*(4), 111–158.
5. World Health Organization—Regional Office for Europe. *Health and social care systems.* http://www.euro.who.int/en/health-topics/Life-stages/healthy-ageing/data-and-statistics/health-and-social-care-systems. Accessed March 15, 2018.
6. Riedel, M., & Kraus, M. (2011). *Informal care provision in Europe: Regulation and profile of providers.* ENEPRI Research Report No. 96, November 2011.
7. Western Sydney University—Centre for Health Research. (2016). *Taking healthcare home.* Ideas Lab Issues Paper.
8. World Health Organization. (2002). Active aging. A policy framework.
9. Bocquaire, E. (2016). *Long-term care coverage in Europe.* https://www.soa.org/Files/Pubs/pub-2016-05-ltc-coverage-europe.pdf. Accessed March 15, 2018.
10. European Association of Service Providers for Persons with Disabilities (EASPD). *Social welfare systems across Europe.* http://www.easpd.eu/sites/default/files/sites/default/files/SensAge/d4-social_welfare_systems_across_europe.pdf. Accessed March 15, 2018.
11. David, S., Sheikh, F., Mahajan, D., Greenough, W., & Bellantoni, M. (2016). Whom do we serve? Describing the target population for post-acute and long-term care, Focusing on nursing facility settings, in the era of population health in the United States. *Journal of the American Medical Directors Association, 17*(7), 574–580.
12. Vrijhoef, H., & Thorlby, R. (2016). *Developing care for a changing population: Supporting patients with costly complex needs.* London: Nuffield Trust.
13. Pla de Salut de Catalunya 2016–2020. (2016). Un sistema centrat en la persona: públic, universal i just. In Catalunya. DdSGd, editor.: Direcció General de Planificació en Salut.
14. Petermans, J., & Piau, A. (2017). Gerontechnology: Don't miss the train, but which is the right carriage? *European Geriatric Medicine, 8*(4), 281–283.
15. Dupuy, L., Froger, C., Consel, C., & Sauzeon, H. (2017). Everyday functioning benefits from an assisted living platform amongst frail older adults and their caregivers. *Frontiers in Aging Neuroscience, 9,* 302.
16. Yusif, S., Soar, J., & Hafeez-Baig, A. (2016). Older people, assistive technologies, and the barriers to adoption: A systematic review. *International Journal of Medical Informatics, 94,* 112–116.
17. Mori, A., Dandi, R., Mazeo, M., Verbicaro, R., & Mercurio, G. (2012). Technological solutions potentially influencing the Future of Long Term Care.
18. Aloulou, H., Mokhtari, M., Tiberghien, T., Biswas, J., Phua, C., Kenneth Lin, J. H., et al. (2013). Deployment of assistive living technology in a nursing home environment: Methods and lessons learned. *BMC Medical Informatics and Decision Making, 13,* 42.
19. Broadbent, E., Tamagawa, R., Patience, A., Knock, B., Kerse, N., Day, K., et al. (2012). Attitudes towards health-care robots in a retirement village. *Australasian Journal on Ageing., 31*(2), 115–120.
20. Gokalp, H., & Clarke, M. (2013). Monitoring activities of daily living of the elderly and the potential for its use in telecare and telehealth: A review. *Telemedicine and e-Health, 19*(12), 910–923.
21. Hansen, L. O., Young, R. S., Hinami, K., Leung, A., & Williams, M. V. (2011). Interventions to reduce 30-day rehospitalization: A systematic review. *Annals of Internal Medicine, 155*(8), 520–528.
22. Haddock, K. S. (1991). Characteristics of effective discharge planning programs for the frail elderly. *Journal of Gerontological Nursing, 17*(7), 10–14.

Chapter 11
Robots in Home Automation and Assistive Environments

By ROBOTNIK, S&C, AVN

Rafael López Tarazón, Román Navarro García, Sofia Aivalioti, Raquel Ventura and Vagelis Mariatos

11.1 Introduction

It is expected to be a rapid evolution of robots integrated into home automation and assistive environments in the coming decades. During this evolution process, there are basic issues that need to be addressed in order to ensure that robots are able to maintain sustainable innovation with the confidence of providers, patients, consumers and investors.[1] There are several drivers that move this development but also technological challenges to overcome. However, the integration is desirable only if it provides a set of benefits, such as a higher quality support, lower cost, adaptability to changing needs of the individual user and long-term support.

[1]Simshaw et al. [1].

R. L. Tarazón (✉) · R. N. García
Robotnik Automation SLL, Valencia, Spain
e-mail: rlopez@robotnik.es

R. N. García
e-mail: rnavarro@robotnik.es

S. Aivalioti · R. Ventura
Sensing & Control S.L., Barcelona, Spain
e-mail: sofia.aivalioti@sensingcontrol.com

R. Ventura
e-mail: raquel.ventura@sensingcontrol.com

V. Mariatos
AVN Innovative Technology Solutions, Limassol, Cyprus
e-mail: emariatos@avntechgroup.com

V. Karkaletsis et al. (eds.), *RADIO–Robots in Assisted Living*,
https://doi.org/10.1007/978-3-319-92330-7_11

11.2 Overview of the Current Situation

With regard to robots in home, there is concern that premature and obtrusive legislation might hamper scientific advancement and prevent potential advantages from happening, burden competitiveness or cause economic or other inefficiencies. At the same time, somehow paradoxically, it is accepted that the lack of a reliable and secure legal environment may equally hinder technological innovation.[2] A transparent regulatory environment is seen as a key element for the development of a robotics and autonomous systems market, where products and services can be incubated and deployed.[3] Currently, there is limited legislation in place that applies to robotics in health care to a greater or lesser extent depending on the type of the robot in question (Table 11.1).

In the absence of specific legislation, the usual point of reference for robots and robotic devices is the International Organization for Standardization and specifically the ISO 13482:2014 standard, which has been developed to specify safety requirements for personal care robots.[4]

The ISO 13482:2014 has been created in recognition of the particular hazards presented by newly emerging robots and robotic devices for new applications in non-industrial environments for providing services rather than manufacturing applications in industrial applications. This international standard focuses on the safety requirements for personal care robots in non-medical applications.

This standard specifies requirements and guidelines for the inherently safe design, protective measures and information for use of personal care robots, in particular, the following three types of personal care robots:

- Mobile servant robot,
- Physical assistant robot and
- Person carrier robot.

11.2.1 Drivers for Robots' Integration in Home Automation and Assistive Environments

- **EU context**

One of the latest trends in Ambient Assisted Living (AAL) technologies receiving active interest from the European research community (e.g. Horizon 2020 research

[2]RoboLaw EU project deliverable, D6.2 Guidelines on Regulating Robotics, published on 22 September 2014.

[3]UK Robotics and Autonomous Systems Special Interest Group (RAS-SIG), 2014:7; cited at ROBOLAW 2014.

[4]Holder et al. [2].

Table 11.1 Related legislation in EU

Regulation	Year	Key points
Health and safety		
Machinery Directive 2006/42/EC	2006	It defines essential health and safety requirements of general application, supplemented by a number of more specific requirements for certain categories of machinery
Defective Product Directive, 85/374/EEC	1985	It establishes the principle that the producer of a product is liable for damages caused by a defect in his product
Data protection and privacy		
Directive 2016/680	2016	It aims to protect natural persons with regard to the processing of personal data by competent authorities for the purposes of the prevention, investigation, detection or prosecution of criminal offences or the execution of criminal penalties, and on the free movement of such data, and repealing Council Framework Decision 2008/977/JHA
Directive 2009/136 amends 2002/58/EC	2009	It contains basic standards aimed at ensuring confidence of users in the services and electronic communications technologies. In particular, aims at the prohibition of 'spam', installation of undesired items (cookies) and ensures security policy with respect to the processing of personal data
ePrivacy Directive 2002/58/EC	2002	It concerns the processing of personal data and the protection of privacy in the electronic communications sector
Data Protection Directive 95/46/EC	1995	It aims to protect individuals with regard to the processing of personal data and on the free movement of such data. The Directive applies to data processed by automated means (e.g. a computer database of customers) and data contained in or intended to be part of non-automated filing systems (traditional paper files)

project calls) helps provisioning daily activities, based on monitoring activities of daily living (ADL) and issuing reminders,[5] as well as helping with mobility and automation.[6] Exploiting novel sensor modality such as video processing, audio processing as well as processing approaches such as fuzzy logic and effective modelling offer enhanced monitoring and control capabilities. Finally, such technologies promote sociability amongst users sharing common interest, activities and hobbies or with their family, friends, doctors and caregivers[7,8] highlighting further the interconnection with Internet of Things (IoT) approaches.

[5]Pollack et al. [3].

[6]Spenko et al. [4].

[7]Mynatt et al. [5].

[8]Vetere et al. [6].

EU identified and highlighted the needs of the increasing ageing European population and they have to be addressed, namely, issues regarding risk of cognitive impairment, frailty and social exclusion with considerable negative consequences for their independence, quality of life, including that of those who care for them and for the sustainability of health and care systems. Special emphasis is given by the EU on the development of robotic services applied in the context of AAL and particularly for supporting ageing population. The key concepts that need to be addressed regard modularity, cost-effectiveness, reliability, flexibility, applicability to realistic settings and acceptability by the end users.

Over the last years, research projects in robotics for ageing well have been funded under the ICT strand of the seventh research framework programme (FP7) and under the AAL Programme, with a total budget of 50 M€. In addition, since 2015, a batch of care robotics projects have been launched under the Horizon 2020 Programme, with a total funding amount of 185 M€.

- **Cloud Technologies**

Cloud computing has become a necessary tool during the last years. The principal functionality is to provide remote computational resources as services invoked through a network.[9] This gives the possibility to provide low-resource devices with access to a massive amount of data and computation power, including distributed and parallel processing. Cloud computing is expanding in several domains and improving in provided services. It offers ease of data exchange, scalability of solutions and flexibility in configuration among others. The robot's connection to the cloud provides the possibility of introducing dynamic machine learning algorithms, collective robot learning offering enhanced capabilities regarding aspects such as speech recognition, emotion recognition and localization.[10]

- **Smart Assistants**

Only a few years ago, the concept of artificial presence (as the one of robots) was considered high risk, as the anticipated acceptance by humans was unknown. Therefore, AAL and smart home architectures focused on the 'de-personalization' of the installation, hiding the interface to the smart infrastructure (and the cloud-based services) under screen-based GUIs. The RADIO project insisted at that time on bringing a partner (the robot) in the scene, taking that risk.

Since then, smart assistants like Apple Siri and Amazon Alexa have entered the market with unprecedented acceptance; rapidly shifting the interface paradigm. Future systems, based on robot-centric access to the smart home and assisted living problems, will leverage from this and add smart assistant interfaces enabling the user to literally talk and interact to his/her robot.

---

[9]Pinta et al. [7].

[10]Pinta et al. [7].

11.2.2 Technological Challenges for the Integration of Robots in Home Automation and Assistive Environments

- **Interoperability**

One of the major challenges for wide adoption of robotics in home automation and assisted living is that of interoperability of various devices. Various sensors, smart appliances, network interfaces, actuators, location devices and the robots need to connect seamlessly at various levels concurrently:

- Network layer—at this level, all nodes should be able to exchange data, either directly or through some bridge or gateway. This can be achieved either by having a single-network installation where all nodes use the same protocols or by ensuring that the multiple networks can connect at the bridge points. Single-network systems are feasible today but they are not growing because (a) the initial setup cost is big and (b) the risk of following a non-future-proof protocol is still high. Industry trends do not show any real convergence; on the contrary, many standardisation initiatives are competing with no clear winner foreseen.
- Semantic layer—at this level (and assuming data transfer is achieved at the network layer), the way this data is constructed and processed has to enable interoperability. Having data semantics defined will allow multiple applications to run in a heterogeneous system, allowing upgrade of the system or provider selection without having to reinstall or reconfigure the infrastructure. Interoperability at this level is not possible today and there is no industry-driven approach to achieve it.

The above points show that achieving an open, configurable and expandable system, which ensures interoperability of devices and applications from various vendors is a major challenge. A challenge, however, has to be confronted by any attempt to develop and deploy a smart home for assisted living. The RADIO consortium tackled interoperability at the network level, by supporting multiple wireless standards.

- **Security**

An important aspect in recent home automation scenarios is the security of the entire system, especially of wireless connections. Therefore, methods have been developed that take this into consideration and are able to face these challenges.

At the wireless infrastructure layers, this is accomplished by employment of the latest security updates in Z-Wave and Bluetooth Low Energy (BLE) standards. At the embedded SW and HW level, all current measures have been taken and any future security updates can be updated on the field. By using reconfigurable architectures, the maintenance of programmable hardware is enabled in so far, as updated security standards can easily be implemented. The RADIO approach is based on the Xilinx Zynq SoC, providing an all programmable approach for both software and hardware. The software part is hereby realised by a modern ARM multi-core processor, while FPGA hardware resembles the programmable and reconfigurable hardware.

- **Heterogeneity of solutions**

The RADIO ecosystem consists of several processing elements, ranging from microcontrollers over processors to FPGAs. The sensors are connected to gateways which are running on an ARM processor. These sensors establish a connection via a microcontroller within the dedicated dongles for either BLE or Z-Wave communication. The RADIO robot consists of two main processing platforms naming the Intel NUC, which is a processor system, and the PicoZed, which is a low-power development board containing the Xilinx Zynq SoC. By using the proposed all programmable hardware, a heterogeneous approach is featured. This applies therefore not only to the diversity of used gateways but also to the processing elements itself. One heterogeneous challenge for the RADIO robot is to incorporate both processing systems to work cooperatively on dedicated robot tasks.

- **Localization**

In order for the robot to be a useful addition in home automation and assistive environments, the robot needs to be autonomous. This is the necessary condition for further technological improvements. Figure 11.1 shows the tasks of the autonomous robot control loop. It consists of localization, cognition, motion control and perception. Each task depends on the prior tasks, and thus all tasks have to be executed continuously. The cognition task requires the data from the location task, i.e. the robot's position in a known environment. From a higher control level, the cognition task receives a goal it needs to achieve. This can be a target position for the robot or an optimal path planning for grabbing an object. The cognition task provides the motion control task with the desired movements to execute in the real-world environment. The motion control task is the only task that interacts with the environment. One problem that needs to be tackled in this task is solving the

Fig. 11.1 The four task phases of an autonomous robot

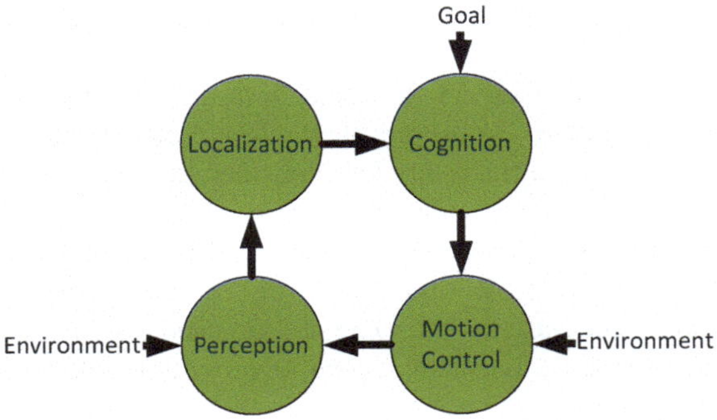

inverse kinematics problem. This is especially important for grabbing objects. The final state of the robot is then sent to the perception task where all sensor data is accumulated and analysed so that the localization task can process this information.

- **High obsolescence rates**

A challenging factor in the field is the product's short life cycle. Robotic technology and ICT products are characterised by high obsolescence rates. For instance, hardware become obsolete in only a few years and are replaced by new ones, while software gets updates at times and it also becomes obsolete and users switch to new ones. In this dynamic context, most of the revenues are generated in the very short run, while there is an increased need for new products and services.

Robots currently are developed and provided by firms that have been used to such short life cycles, originating from the personal computer/laptop or from the—even shorter—software marketplaces. For robots to be successful, their life cycle model should resemble that of white appliances or even cars, ensuring that the individual's investment is justified in terms of return.

- **Energy consumption**

The proposed hardware architectures enable the low-power operation of the robot. Therefore, a camera is connected to the PicoZed which analyses the scenery and wakes up the power-hungry components of the robot, such as the Intel NUC and the processing core of the PicoZed itself. The BLE technology used within the RADIO approach allows the low-power operation by design, thus allowing long operation times and availability of the RADIO ecosystem. As the RADIO ecosystem also includes Z-Wave devices, which are not as power-hungry as Ethernet-based components, further steps towards energy-efficient homes have been taken within the RADIO projects.

11.2.3 Initial Roadmap for the Integration of Robots in Home Automation and Assistive Environments

The main technological advancement of RADIO is the combination of cutting-edge technologies that enable high-quality systems that meet human-centric requirements by being adaptive, interactive and contextual. This high-level concept is translated into specific technological challenges that need to be addressed.

- **Communication systems**

These systems are composed of a number of different devices that require a fast interaction between them in order to share information. Robust communication systems are required to enable interactive solutions. For example, the robot requires proper WiFi connection to navigate inside a house in order to be continuously connected to the global controllers. Robotic platform is expected to support two communication interfaces. On the one hand, it is required to support a communication with the sensors gathering environmental information (laser, RGBD cameras, microphones, etc.), while on the other hand the robot must be able to interact with the RADIO home controller in order to access services external to the RADIO home. Physical connection between the mobile robot and smart home devices and the RADIO home controller must be achieved through WiFi connection to the ADSL router that also provides Internet connectivity. An off-the-shelf WiFi sub-dongle will suffice for such connectivity requirement.

- **Navigation, localisation**

There are many handicaps that robots find when navigating in unstructured home environments, like pushing away obstacles, using stairs or elevators, sidestepping humans, pets, other robots, etc. They all require 3D perception and the use of cameras (cameras are cheaper and can be richer in information than many LIDAR sensors). RGBD sensors are great for indoors; they are cheap and we can use them to map with different approaches (i.e. real-time SLAM software for RGBD sensors) with many functions such as multi-session mapping, appearance-based closure detection, map optimization to new constraints, 2D projected map, etc.[11] The house needs to have a clear path for the navigation of the robot: the robotic platform must be always able to locate a path to move. It is important not to drop obstacles that might cause difficulty in robot movement.

- **Human–Machine Interaction (HMI)**

The integration of robots in home automation and assistive environments require some improvements in the design of elderly HMI. Effective end user involvement in all stages of the system development is highly desired. Creative design activities and evaluation methods that suit the elderly need to keep improving. User interfaces through television, touchscreen, avatars or speech have shown significant acceptability for the elderly. Television allows displaying avatars that they are used to show exercise or reminder messages. Also, the usage of television as the main interaction device is possible using arrow buttons of the remote control for navigation.

- **Robotics technology**

The healthcare community requires low-cost robotic aid that provides input–output capabilities to the user interface, control, safety and autonomy procedures. For example, once the robot detects that its battery is low, it goes directly to the recharging station, in a similar way as the vacuum cleaner robots. User's acceptability depends on physical structure of the mobile robot, interaction, mobility systems, system of sensors such as cameras, infrared, shared control, etc.

---

[11]In order to cope with the navigation and localization problem, RADIO makes use of ROS since it provides powerful and well-tested software to deal with navigation issues. Gmapping and hector slam are the most used ROS packages by the community for SLAM (both based in MCL).

- **Artificial Intelligence**

With the emergence of sensors that keep getting better, smaller and more capable of measuring almost anything, context awareness will be a key factor for most applications in home automatization and assistive environments. The availability of many types of sensors in smartphones and the IoT are providing enormous volumes of contextual data available. This has serious implications for Artificial Intelligence (AI). First, it is expected that systems are self-aware and understand the context through reasoning process. The systems are trained for specific contexts and then use contextual reasoning and specific learning techniques to efficiently and effectively solve problems. Context reasoning is as important as learning for deriving models. The next AI advances should find a way to balance contextual reasoning and machine learning that enable systems to be dynamic enough to adapt and improve with experience. Second, AI plays a relevant role in acquiring contextual awareness through the use of speech understanding mechanisms and emotion recognition by face and voice detection.

- **Security, Privacy and Data Protection**

Security, privacy and data protection are critical issues in the IoT domain when this involves users who store and exchange their medical data. The aforementioned legislation provides guidelines regarding the use of personal data retrieved from ICT technologies (ePrivacy Directive) in order to avoid misuse. A safe approach suggests the use of data encryption and digital certificate infrastructure for ensuring confidentiality and integrity of the medical data collected from wearables, sensors.[12] A secure transmission to the cloud and access to official and unofficial caregivers is also important.

- **Technology Standards and Specifications**

Technology standards and specifications provide the basis to achieve interoperability, integration and scalability through standardised protocols and data models. The standards should apply to all technologies, robotic, wireless sensor networks, health monitoring devices, smart home systems, etc.

11.3 Market Opportunities Arisen from RADIO Robot

The RADIO outcomes that can generate market opportunities are the next:

- Audiovisual Activities of Daily Living (ADL) detection methods: Methods that detect ADL from audio and visual signal.

---

[12]Doukas [8].

- ROS/IoT middleware integration: Integration of Robot OS components with IoT middleware and web services and with human–robot interaction components for integrated automation/mobile robot environments.
- Privacy-preserving Data Mining: Data management components for privacy-preserving data mining.
- WSN gateway design and development: Enhanced WSN gateway supporting heterogeneous communication technologies both concerning the WSN network and the back-end communication. Additionally, respective design offers advanced functional features and resilience characteristics incorporating internal databases and intelligence.
- BLE communication technologies: Enhance BLE enabling extended coverage area, mobility support, dynamic topology support and more efficient traffic/data management.
- Design and develop an end-to-end versatile communication platform: The proposed platform (ATLAS) is able to be easily extended and expanded concerning various critical aspects. Particular focus has been devoted to offering flexible interfaces, allowing the easy integration of future communication technologies. Additionally, support of all prominent database types is offered, delivering advanced performance characteristics. Finally, the development of application is significantly facilitated following the microservice paradigm, allowing the easy plugging and unplugging of specific application components. In the context of RADIO, it is used for various functionalities intended for the technical personnel.
- ADL detection methods through smart home sensors: Data mining and machine learning techniques will be developed to detect ADLs through the energy consumption in homes. Each activity is associated with measurable features such as the time of day, users' movement patterns through the space and the on/off status of various electrical appliances.
- Advance TurtleBot2 platform to support RADIO services: Adapting the generic platform of TurtleBot2 to carry hardware equipment that supports RADIO services.
- Hardware acceleration for intensive audio and visual processing: To achieve increased autonomy of the robot, power-efficient solutions are developed by the development of dedicated and highly parameterised IPs implemented in hardware that enable processing of audio and video at lower power and higher speeds.
- Hardware acceleration architecture (Based on the Xilinx tool flow): The image processing algorithms that need to be accelerated require a specific architecture in order for them to be integrated into the ROS environment of the robot.
- APIs for the connection between controller, robot and smart home: The controller module will be in charge of getting information from the different platforms, robot and smart home, combining and analysing data to create the proper ADLs. This requires a direct connection between the controller and smart home and controller and robot through APIs.

- RADIO complete architecture and services: From an elder care facility, RADIO complete architecture will provide new opportunities to hospitalisation. It will also offer to caregivers and nurses remote patient monitoring and after a surgical intervention, it will offer rehabilitation before going back to their homes.

11.4 Conclusion

As we have seen throughout this chapter, the usage of robots integrated into home automation and assistive environments is not 100% solved from some perspectives:

- Although integration is technically feasible with the existing and emerging technologies, there are still some technological difficulties and challenges that must be solved (as interoperability, security and heterogeneity of solutions or energy consumption).
- There is still work needed for enhancing standardisation options and elaborate suitable legislation in order to adapt to the changing needs and technology advancements.
- User's acceptability will be the key aspect of the commercialization and therefore these technologies have to cover real needs and offer the appropriate return on investment.

Finally, we can summarise the next steps as the key points to commercialise the RADIO solution:

- Establish a robust communication system to enable interactive solutions.
- The robot should have a localization and navigation system.
- Address user's need for continuously improving systems for human–machine interaction.
- Ensure user's acceptability of robot's design, data collection, behaviour and functionalities.
- AI to provide a dynamic service adapting and improving with experience.
- Provide security, privacy and data protection.
- Comply with technology standards and specifications.

References

1. Simshaw, D., Terry, N., Hauser, K., & Cummings, M. (2016). Regulating healthcare robots: maximizing opportunities while minimizing risks. *Richmond Journal of Law and Technology, 22*(3). https://hal.pratt.duke.edu/sites/hal.pratt.duke.edu/files/u13/REGULATING%20HEALTHCARE%20ROBOTS.pdf.

2. Holder, C., Khurana, V., Harrison, F., & Jacobs, L. (2016). Robotics and law: Key legal and regulatory implications of the robotics age (Part I of II). *Computer Law & Security Review, 32*, 383–402.
3. Pollack, M. E., Brown, L., Colbry, D., McCarthy, C. E., Orosz, C., Peintner, B., et al. (2003). Autominder: An intelligent cognitive orthotic system for people with memory impairment. In *Proceedings of Robotic Autonomous Systems*.
4. Spenko, M., et al. (2006). Pamm—A robotic aid to the elderly for mobility assistance and monitorng for the elderly. *Transactions on Neural System Rehabilitation*.
5. Mynatt, E. D., Rowan, J., Jacobs, A., & Craighill, S. (2001). Digital family portraits: Supporting peace of mind for extended family members. In *Proceedings of SIGCHI Conference on Human Factors in Computing Systems*.
6. Vetere, F., Davis, H., Gibbs, M., & Howard, S. (2009). The magic box and collage: Responding to the challenge of distributed intergenerational play. *Journal of Human-Computer Studies*.
7. Pinta, D. L. P. J., Maestre Torreblanca, J. M., Jurado, I., & Reyes De Cozar, S. (2017). Off the shelf cloud robotics for the smart home: Empowering a wireless robot through cloud computing. *Sensors, 17*, 525. https://doi.org/10.3390/s17030525.
8. Doukas, C. (2012). Enabling data protection through PKI encryption in IoT M-Health devices. In *Proceedings of the 12th International Conference on Bioinformatics and Bioengineering (BIBE), Larnaca, Cyprus* (pp. 25–29), November 11–13, 2012.

Index

V. Karkaletsis et al. (eds.), *RADIO–Robots in Assisted Living*,
https://doi.org/10.1007/978-3-319-92330-7

The manufacturer's authorised representative in the EU is Springer Nature Customer Service Centre GmbH, Europaplatz 3, 69115 Heidelberg, Germany. If you have any concerns regarding our products, please contact ProductSafety@springernature.com

Printed and bound by CPI Group (UK) Ltd, Croydon, CR0 4YY
05/10/2026
02228122-0003